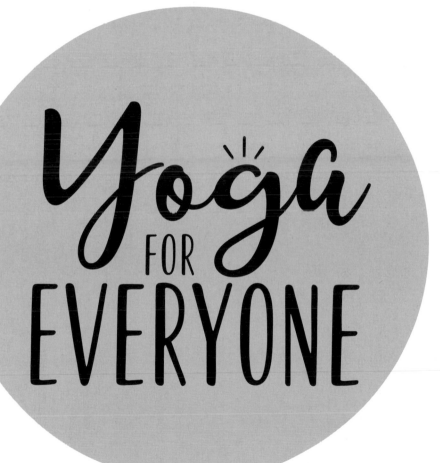

Yoga
FOR
EVERYONE

Yoga
FOR
EVERYONE
50 POSES FOR EVERY TYPE OF BODY

>>> DIANNE BONDY <<<

ALPHA

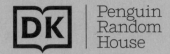

Publisher Mike Sanders
Editor Christopher Stolle
Senior Designer Jessica Lee
Art Director Nigel Wright
Photographer Joanna Wojewoda
Proofreader Lisa Starnes
Indexer Brad Herriman

First American Edition, 2019
Published in the United States by DK Publishing
6081 E. 82nd Street, Indianapolis, Indiana 46250

Copyright © 2019 Dorling Kindersley Limited
DK, a Division of Penguin Random House LLC
21 22 10 9 8 7 6 5
006–312956–APRIL/2019

Note: This publication contains the opinions and ideas of its author(s). It is intended to provide helpful and
informative material on the subject matter covered. It is sold with the understanding that the author(s) and
publisher are not engaged in rendering professional services in the book. If the reader requires personal
assistance or advice, a competent professional should be consulted. The author(s) and publisher specifically
disclaim any responsibility for any liability, loss, or risk, personal or otherwise, which is incurred as a
consequence, directly or indirectly, of the use and application of
any of the contents of this book.

Trademarks: All terms mentioned in this book that are known to be or are suspected of being trademarks or
service marks have been appropriately capitalized. Alpha Books, DK, and Penguin Random House LLC cannot
attest to the accuracy of this information. Use of a term in this book should not be regarded as affecting the
validity of any trademark or service mark.

A catalog record for this book
is available from the Library of Congress.
ISBN 978-1-4654-8077-4
Library of Congress Catalog Number: 2018958035

DK books are available at special discounts when purchased in bulk for sales promotions, premiums, fundraising,
or educational use. For details, contact: DK Publishing Special Markets, 1450 Broadway, Suite 801, New York,
NY 10018
SpecialSales@dk.com

Printed and bound in China

Photo Credits: Cover 123RF.com: Liliia Rudchenko / rudchenko; Cover, 2-3 Dreamstime.com: Shakila Malavige
All other images © Dorling Kindersley Limited
For further information see: www.dkimages.com

A WORLD OF IDEAS:
SEE ALL THERE IS TO KNOW

www.dk.com

Contents

FOREWORD

I remember the first time I stepped into a yoga class. I sat in my car until I was almost late for class. My heart was racing as I unrolled a mat in the back corner of the class. I didn't know the first thing about yoga. But I was pretty sure that people like me didn't belong in a yoga studio.

You see, I'm plus-sized. A person in a bigger body. Round. Fat. (You can pick the word you like.) This big body has always been my "yoga body." Yoga marketing and the covers of magazines had taught me that only thin, wealthy, hyperflexible, white women practiced yoga, and so there I was in my fat, awkward, tattooed body and my decidedly unfashionable workout clothing, nervous and waiting for class to start.

I struggled through that first class, but I felt such a profound benefit from the internal regulation tools that yoga offered me that I kept coming back. After each class, my mind was quieter, I was less self-conscious, I felt more grounded in my body. But that doesn't mean the physical practice of yoga felt easy to me.

When I began practicing yoga, teachers didn't know what the heck to do with me. Even though my body wasn't making many of the shapes they were asking of it, in most of the classes I went to, I was ignored. Teachers didn't offer me modifications, variations on poses, or ways to personalize my practice. Sometimes, teachers would tell me to "use a prop if I needed one," but I was clueless about what to do with props.

Looking back now, being ignored for a few years of my practice was a gift because it meant I had to be creative and have agency when it came to my practice. Back then, there weren't online videos telling you how to modify poses. There weren't yogis who looked like me with hundreds of thousands of followers on Instagram. And in class, no one was telling me why I couldn't step my foot forward between my hands to get from Downward Dog into Lunge or how to get there in a different way, so I had to figure it out myself.

Back then, I'd have given anything for a book like this—or a teacher like Dianne. She's a masterful

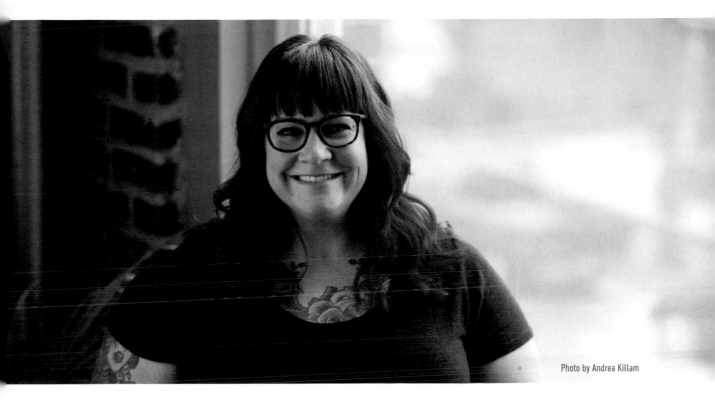

teacher and has an intuitive understanding of what folks' bodies are capable of. That's why she's the perfect person to write *Yoga for Everyone*.

Each pose in this book shows several different ways to personalize and adapt the traditional expression of a posture. This gives folks in many different body types — people of all shapes, sizes, and abilities — the opportunity to receive the benefits of each pose, even if they don't look like someone on the cover of a yoga magazine.

Yoga for Everyone shows representations of what the human beings who practice yoga actually look like. Contrary to what media images would have you believe, yoga isn't just for thin, wealthy, flexible, white women. Wellness belongs to all of us. Wellness is our birthright. Flipping through these pages, you'll surely see someone you can identify with and you'll definitely find a version of each yoga pose that can work for your unique human body.

Dianne's teachings will give you agency to personalize your practice. You don't need to change who you are or hope for some magical day when your body is thinner, younger, fitter, or more flexible. In the words of Arthur Ashe: "Start where you are. Use what you have. Do what you can."

Learning to personalize my yoga practice all those years ago helped me make peace with my body. I became more physically fluent—and that changed everything. Mindful movement made me more certain of myself. My body got stronger. I learned to move with intention. And I also made friends with my mind.

My yoga practice helped me feel sure—helped me know in my bones—that my body was a powerful, good, and safe place to be.

Yoga for Everyone can also help you learn that. Your body is powerful, good, and a safe place to be — just as it is today.

AMBER KARNES
Founder, Body Positive Yoga
bodypositiveyoga.com

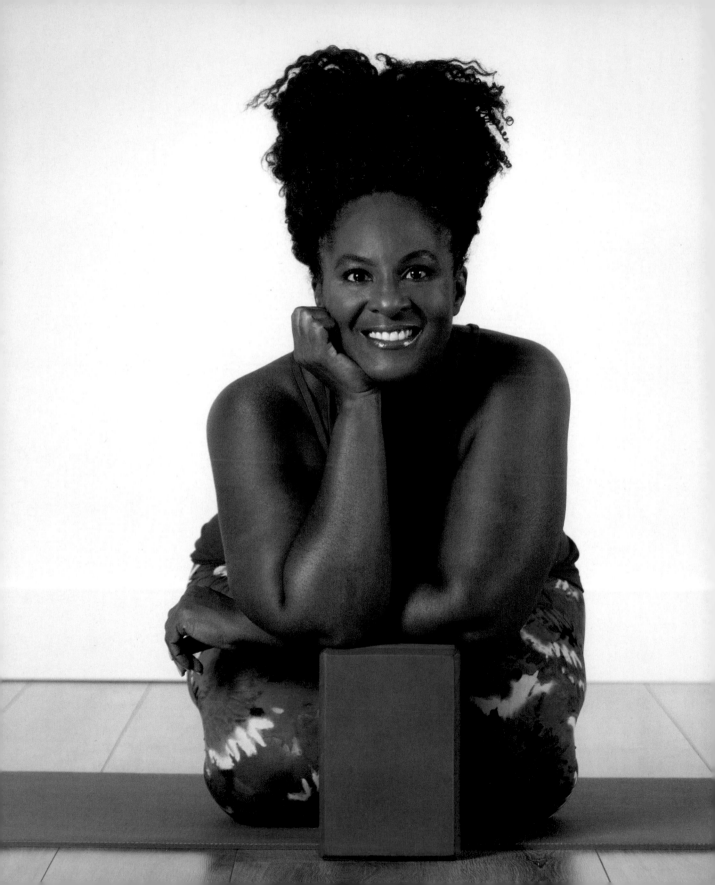

Yes, You Can Do Yoga!

I began practicing yoga when I was a young girl. My mother practiced yoga as a way to cope with the stress of being a new mom in a new place. We practiced together at home and it became a special moment for us. Yoga is one of the greatest gifts my mother gave to me. Yoga taught me courage, compassion, connection—and how to do a handstand.

Over the course of my life, I've practiced, studied, and taught many different styles of yoga. As a woman of color in a more substantial body, I often felt like I didn't belong in the practice. My body didn't move the same way as smaller bodies, and because of this, I had a number of physical and emotional challenges in public classes. I didn't move as quickly as others. Yoga began to feel like an exclusionary club for the wealthy, thin, flexible, or able-bodied. No one looked like me or moved like me—and I felt left out.

As I struggled to learn yoga poses, I began to understand that not all bodies move in the same way. Poses look different in different bodies and we need to make space for this. Poses like the Warrior series, Downward Dog, and Tree all take on a different shape and orientation in different-sized bodies. We must allow for the individualization of each pose to accommodate different abilities. It thus became my passion to share what I've learned during my 25 years of teaching yoga and movement to bodies of all shapes, sizes, and levels of ability.

This book intends to provide you with the tools you need to begin a customized yoga practice with adaptations that work for your body. You'll find the basic movements for many classic yoga poses as well as a variety of accessible variations. While this book can help you develop a sustainable at-home practice, it's also beneficial to visit a public yoga class. Practicing with others can provide a great sense of community. And this book can help you develop the confidence to practice in a public setting regardless of whether the other students look or move like you do.

My hope for you is that this book provides you with the tools you need to adapt your practice to your body—no matter where you practice. Most of all, I hope it inspires you to be kind and gentle with your body. It's my belief that a yoga practice can be a catalyst for positive and lasting change.

I wish you the gifts of self-awareness and compassion and the realization that you're more than enough—just as you are.

I dedicate this book to anyone who has felt left out or felt marginalized by this practice. Yoga is for you. You can do this. Let me show you how.

DIANNE BONDY

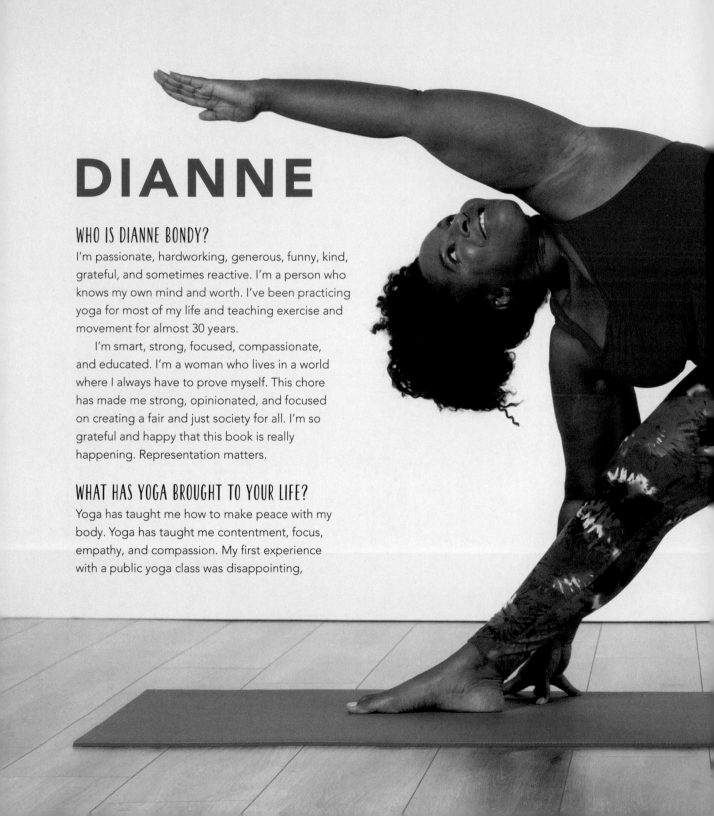

DIANNE

WHO IS DIANNE BONDY?

I'm passionate, hardworking, generous, funny, kind, grateful, and sometimes reactive. I'm a person who knows my own mind and worth. I've been practicing yoga for most of my life and teaching exercise and movement for almost 30 years.

I'm smart, strong, focused, compassionate, and educated. I'm a woman who lives in a world where I always have to prove myself. This chore has made me strong, opinionated, and focused on creating a fair and just society for all. I'm so grateful and happy that this book is really happening. Representation matters.

WHAT HAS YOGA BROUGHT TO YOUR LIFE?

Yoga has taught me how to make peace with my body. Yoga has taught me contentment, focus, empathy, and compassion. My first experience with a public yoga class was disappointing,

FAVORITE POSE
>>> TRIANGLE

MOST CHALLENGING POSE
>>> LOW PLANK

OCCUPATION
>>> YOGA INSTRUCTOR AND BODY POSITIVITY ADVOCATE

which inspired me to open my own space. I attempt to do a 15-minute meditation and yoga practice every day. I use my yoga to navigate the world with peace, kindness, and passion. I love how yoga slows down time. Yoga helps me deal with stress and makes me more aware. I also love the peace of mind and the challenge to my body, and I love feeling a sense of peace and gratitude through movement.

WHAT ADVICE DO YOU HAVE FOR POTENTIAL YOGA PRACTITIONERS?

Start with a beginner in a safe and comfortable environment, like a community center or an online source. Find a teacher who knows how to work with your body and take a chance. I think seeing people who look like you doing yoga will inspire people to try. Seeing all kinds of bodies as yoga bodies is so important.

CHAPTER 1

Yoga Basics

This chapter can help kick-start your yoga practice,
highlighting the benefits of yoga, breathing techniques,
equipment you need, how to set up your own yoga space,
and how to navigate the rest of this book.

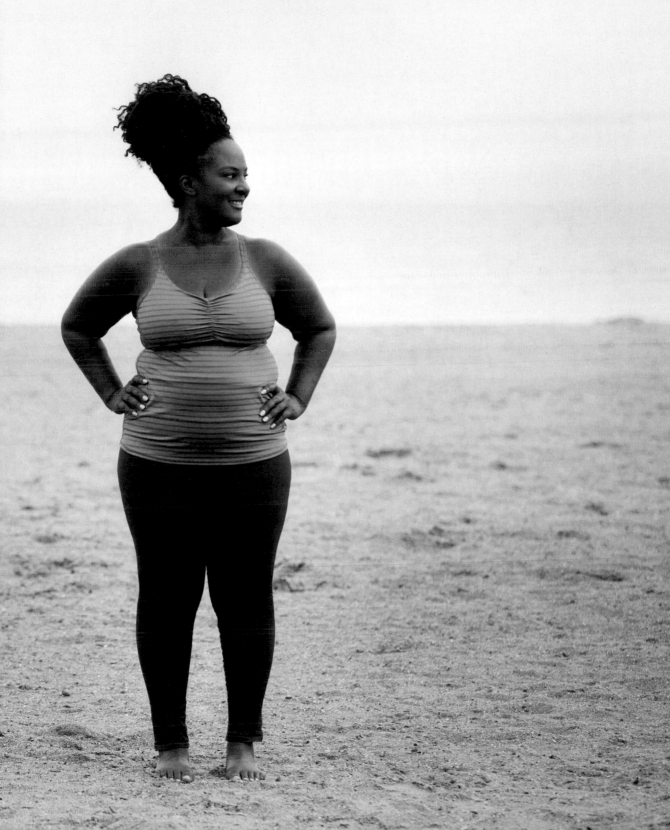

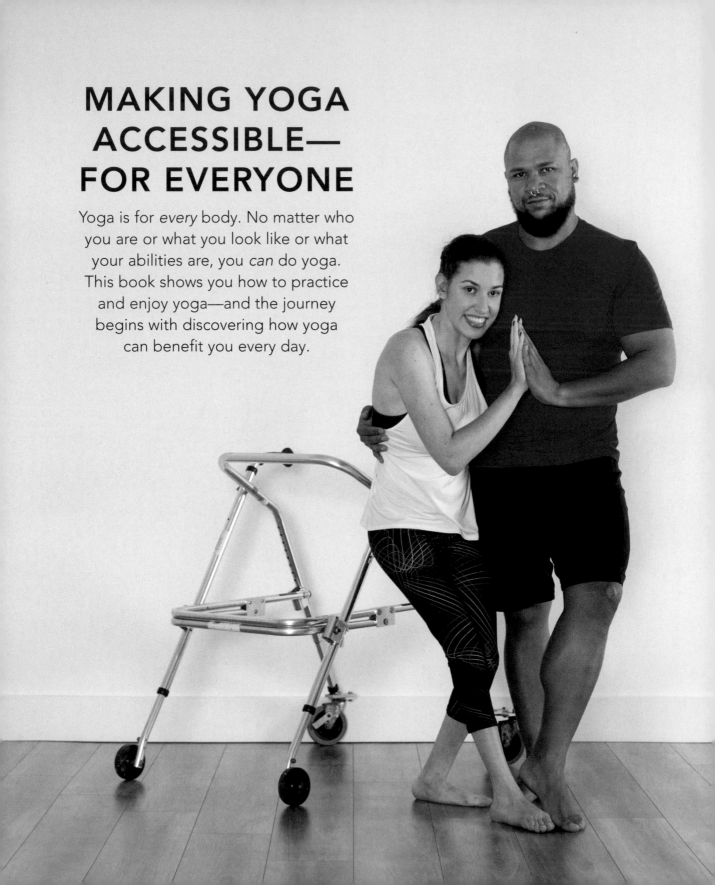

MAKING YOGA ACCESSIBLE—FOR EVERYONE

Yoga is for *every* body. No matter who you are or what you look like or what your abilities are, you *can* do yoga. This book shows you how to practice and enjoy yoga—and the journey begins with discovering how yoga can benefit you every day.

"Yoga is the journey of the self, through the self, to the self."

— EXCERPT FROM *BHAGAVAD GITA*

CREATE VARIATIONS AND ADAPTATIONS

One great reason to appreciate yoga is that any pose can be adapted and varied to suit your needs. Even the most vigorous- and rigorous-looking poses can be tamed to fit your ability. Every pose in this book has at least two variations, giving you a chance to practice poses that might have felt intimidating before. In this way, yoga conforms to you and your needs—and you won't have to skip any poses. You'll develop the confidence to take what you gain from your yoga practice off the mat and into the world around you.

INCREASE PHYSICAL HEALTH

More and more people have begun to discover the powerful influence yoga can have on their bodies. When you practice a pose, you're stretching muscles, helping you strengthen weak areas, further develop strong areas, and potentially prevent injuries. Yoga is also a helpful tool for an aging body. As you get older, your balance, focus, and flexibility begin to diminish. Yoga can help keep you mobile by improving circulation and stability, managing blood pressure, and reducing the risk of heart disease.

RELIEVE STRESS AND PAIN

Most people come to yoga to relieve back pain, increase flexibility, reduce stress, or improve physical and mental health. People often begin a yoga practice simply as another form of movement or exercise, but over time, the practice evolves into a journey of self-exploration. Yoga offers a unique connection between the mind and the spirit. A regular yoga practice can elevate your understanding of self-actualization.

DEVELOP MENTAL ACUITY

Yoga depends as much on your breathing as anything physical. Proper breathing can turn a simple exercise regime into a mindful and transformative experience that leads to greater self-awareness. The philosophies behind yoga can foster body positivity by helping you realize that you're enough. The central tenets of yoga include nonviolence, contentment, gratitude, and self-study. When you practice these actions, you can start to reduce negative self-chatter and allow yourself to believe how amazing you are.

APPRECIATE YOUR BODY

When you apply kindness and compassion to how you move and connect with your body, you can begin to cultivate self-acceptance. Yoga actually invites you to expand your understanding of your body's natural limits, allowing you to make peace with your body as you move on your mat. Yes, negative body image is an invasive issue in Western culture, and social and economic landscapes profit from body dissatisfaction. You're fed a daily stream of unrealistic images of how your body should look and perform, and this creates many issues that directly affect your mental and physical health. But when you practice yoga often, you and your body develop power and influence over your everyday life.

CREATING YOUR PRACTICE

If you're new to yoga, please know this: You can practice anywhere. If you can't make it to a yoga studio or would prefer to practice in private, setting up a home practice gives you the freedom to practice for as long or as short as desired. This is also a great way to keep your practice consistent and sustainable. Because yoga is meant to help reduce stress and create peace of mind, try these suggestions to help you cultivate your practice.

MAKE TIME

Your yoga practice doesn't need to be 90 minutes long every single day. You can start small, doing a pose or two a day, and work toward performing more when you're ready. You don't even need to perform yoga during a single period of time. If you incorporate moments of yoga and meditation throughout your day, you'll find opportunities to practice when you least expect them—and you'll be more willing to practice more often.

SET AN INTENTION

If you're looking to make your yoga practice a regular part of your everyday life, start by setting an intention to get moving! Setting an intention is essentially a built-in measure of accountability. Your intention acts as motivation—the "why" behind your actions. It's up to you to work toward that goal.

CREATE A SPACE

You don't need a lot of space in which to perform yoga. All you really need is enough room for your yoga mat, any props, and your body. One way to make your practice consistent is to choose a convenient spot you walk by every day. You can even place yoga mats in several strategic spots in your dwelling, greatly increasing the likelihood you'll perform yoga every day.

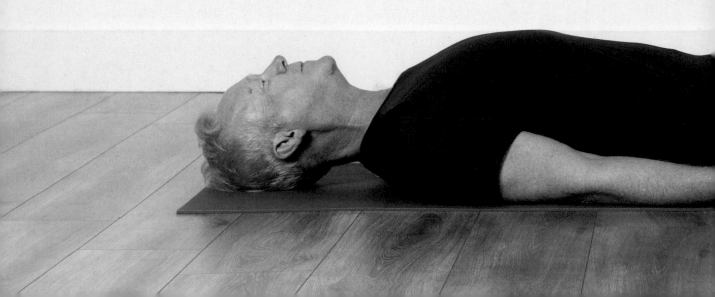

"The success of yoga does not lie in the ability to perform postures but in how it positively changes the way we live our life and our relationships."

— T. K. V. DESIKACHAR, YOGA TEACHER

PRACTICE WHAT YOU LOVE

You don't have to practice all the poses and sequences in this book. Find ones you think you'll enjoy and practice them when you feel like it. In time, you might decide to try poses that initially intimidated you. Make yoga your oasis away from stress and obligation. Create a fun playlist and set aside some time to move your body in all directions. Most importantly, don't beat yourself up if you don't practice for several days, weeks, or months. When you do return to your practice, start slowly again, doing only what feels right to you, and you'll find you haven't missed a step.

FIND YOUR PRACTICE

This book can help you discover how yoga works for you and which poses work for you. You might find that a variation for stability works well with one pose but not for another or that a variation to help with your challenges with mobility doesn't work for you. In these cases, make your own modifications as needed—or just forego a pose, variation, or sequence entirely. Listen to your body and pay attention to how it reacts. You can always revisit a skipped pose in the future. Because yoga is for every body—and that means you!—change your practice to make it what you need it to be for you.

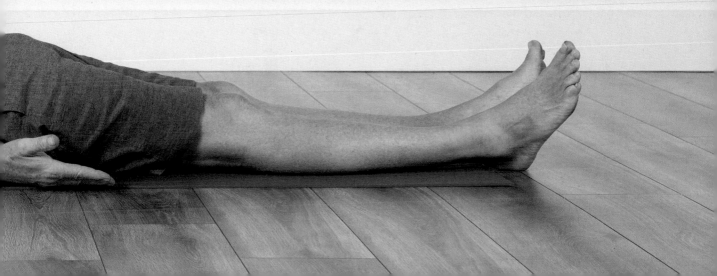

BREATHING TECHNIQUES

Practicing pranayama—the Sanskrit word for breath control—can help you balance your energy, calm your nervous system, and encourage a meditative state. There are three main types of breathing techniques you can explore in your yoga practice —and each one has a different purpose.

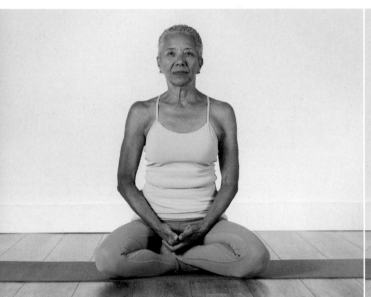 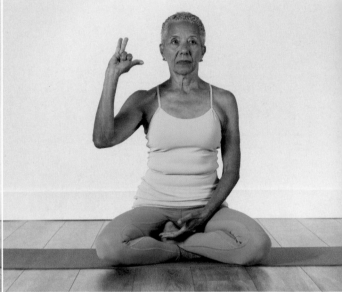

NADI SHODHANA PRANAYAMA

Nadi shodhana—also known as the alternate nostril breath—is a technique you can perform before or after practicing yoga. It brings balance to both sides of your body, helping reduce stress and anxiety, lower your heart rate and blood pressure, relieve tension, and revitalize a tired mind and body. Using the above photos as guides, follow these steps to perform nadi shodhana:

1. Sit on the mat or on a meditation cushion in a comfortable cross-legged position, with your hands resting on your thighs or relaxed at your sides.

2. Bend the index and middle fingers of your right hand toward your right palm and press your right thumb against your right nostril to seal it.

3. Deeply inhale through your left nostril.

4. Seal off your left nostril with your right ring finger and release your right nostril.

5. Deeply exhale through your right nostril.

6. Deeply inhale through your right nostril.

7. Seal off your right nostril with your right thumb and release your left nostril.

8. Deeply exhale through your left nostril. This completes one round of breathing. Repeat these steps for 1 minute or for as long as desired.

UJJAYI PRANAYAMA

Ujjayi—also known as victory breath or ocean breath—is the most common breathing technique used during a yoga practice. It can add texture and

"Master your breath, let the self be in bliss, contemplate on the sublime within you."

— TIRUMALAI KRISHNAMACHARYA, YOGA TEACHER

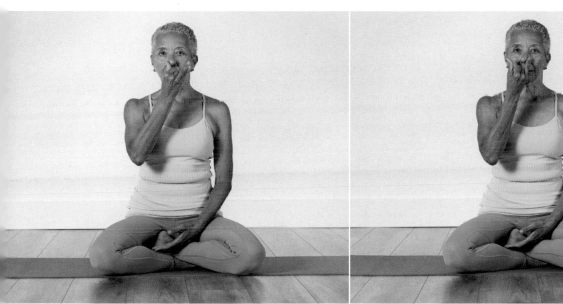 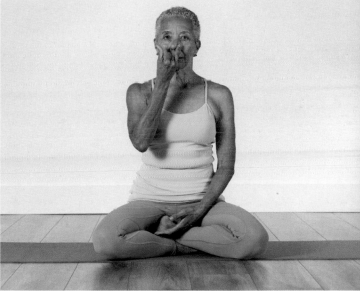

dimension to your breathing pattern, and it heats the body from within and draws life energy upward. Follow these steps to perform ujjayi during the poses in this book:

1. With your mouth closed, inhale a long breath through your nose, gently constrict the back of your throat, and make a subtle *haaah* or *ahhhh* sound.
2. Continue to keep your mouth closed as you exhale a long breath through your nose, continuing to constrict the back of your throat.
3. Repeat these steps throughout each pose.

SAMA VRITTI PRANAYAMA

Sama vritti—also known as square breathing—is an excellent technique for helping relieve stress and reduce anxiety. This method helps refocus your thoughts and bring peace of mind and calm to your entire body. Because of its simplicity, this technique also helps create more space for relaxation in a busy schedule. You can perform this before, during, or after a yoga practice. Follow these steps to perform sama vritti:

1. Deeply inhale for a count of 4 and hold this inhalation for another count of 4. As you inhale, imagine your breath following each side of a square.
2. Deeply exhale for a count of 4 and hold this exhalation for another count of 4. As you exhale, imagine your breath following each side of a square.
3. Repeat these steps for as long as desired or repeat these steps throughout each pose.

WHAT YOU NEED TO PRACTICE YOGA

Props are tools you can use to customize your yoga practice. They can add support, stability, resistance, the opportunity for creativity, and access. They can also allow you to experiment with different movements in poses. This is a brief introduction to the props used in this book.

YOGA MATS

Although a standard yoga mat is 24 inches by 68 inches, you have other options: a longer or wider mat, a stickier mat to prevent slipping, or a thick mat for additional cushioning. If you plan to practice regularly, invest in a high-quality yoga mat.

BLOCKS

Blocks come in a variety of sizes, shapes, and textures, and they provide weight, structure, and stability. They're helpful for many different poses. Have a few different kinds handy to help you customize your practice.

BOLSTERS

Like blocks, bolsters also come in different sizes, shapes, and textures, but they're softer than blocks and provide better support. Find one that feels comfortable when you hug it to your chest.

BLANKETS

A yoga blanket provides better customization and support than a towel. Find one with some weight to it—like ones that are a mix of wool and polyester or Mexican blankets—to allow for extended wear.

STRAPS

Buy a strap that's at least 10 feet long and has the metal D-rings to allow you to adjust the length as needed. Straps that are too long can be difficult to use. If you find that a strap is hard to hold, you can also use a belt, necktie, dog leash, sash, or scarf.

WALL

This is the easiest prop because you can find a wall anywhere. A wall offers accessibility, stabilization, and resistance—and can even aid in relaxation. Use one with plenty of nearby floor space.

CHAIR

If you have limited mobility or flexibility, a chair has especially good versatility. A chair can help you stand or offer support for extended periods of time. A chair can also help you defy gravity by making it easier to go upside down. A simple chair with just a seat and a back is best for yoga practice.

CLOTHES

You should wear clothes that allow you to move freely and without constriction. What matters most is that you feel comfortable no matter what you wear.

"The body is the prop for the soul. So why not let the body be propped by a wall or a block?"

— B. K. S. IYENGAR, YOGA TEACHER

HOW TO USE THIS BOOK

This book has four main components.

STEP-BY-STEP INSTRUCTIONS
FOR PERFORMING POSES

INSTRUCTIONS FOR
MAKING MODIFICATIONS

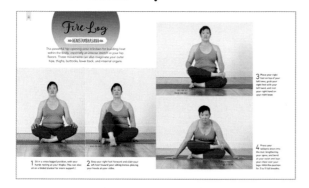

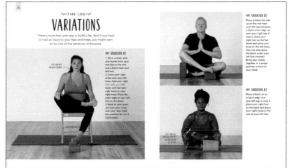

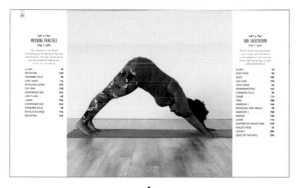

INSTRUCTIONS FOR
PERFORMING YOGA FLOWS

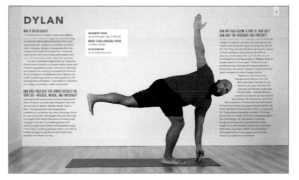

PERSONAL PERSPECTIVES
FROM EACH MODEL

MEET THE MODELS

**DIANNE
BONDY**

READ HER STORY
ON PAGE 10.

**DYLAN
GALOS**

READ HIS STORY
ON PAGE 90.

**JOSIE
DONATO**

READ HER STORY
ON PAGE 56.

**JOHN
AZLEN**

READ HIS STORY
ON PAGE 212.

**GAIL
PARKER**

READ HER STORY
ON PAGE 238.

**DON
COYLE**

READ HIS STORY
ON PAGE 158.

**ALEX
TRAUBERT**

READ HER STORY
ON PAGE 124.

**GWEN
JFUN**

READ HER STORY
ON PAGE 186.

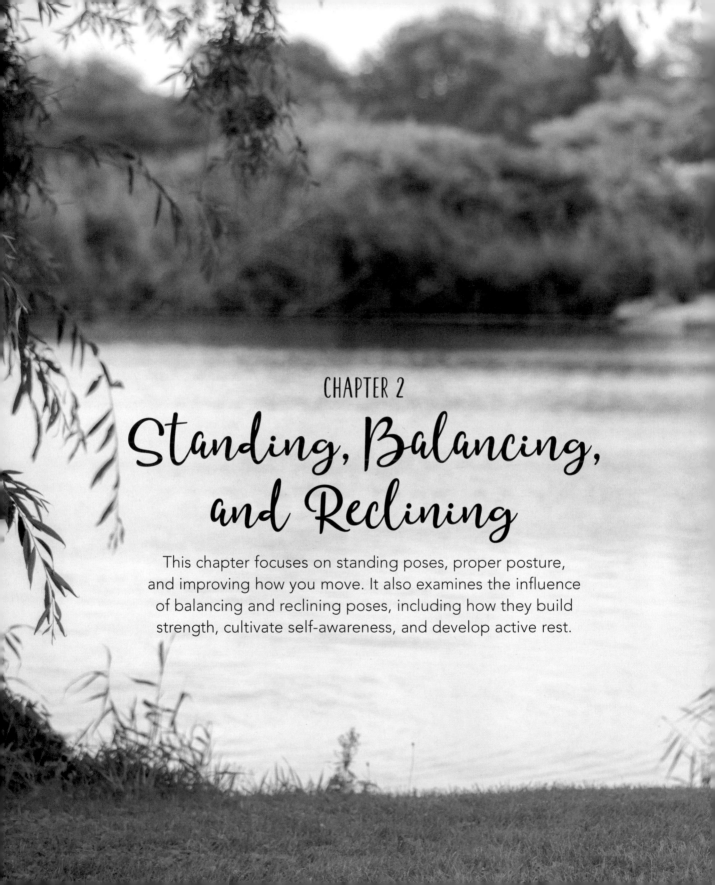

CHAPTER 2

Standing, Balancing, and Reclining

This chapter focuses on standing poses, proper posture, and improving how you move. It also examines the influence of balancing and reclining poses, including how they build strength, cultivate self-awareness, and develop active rest.

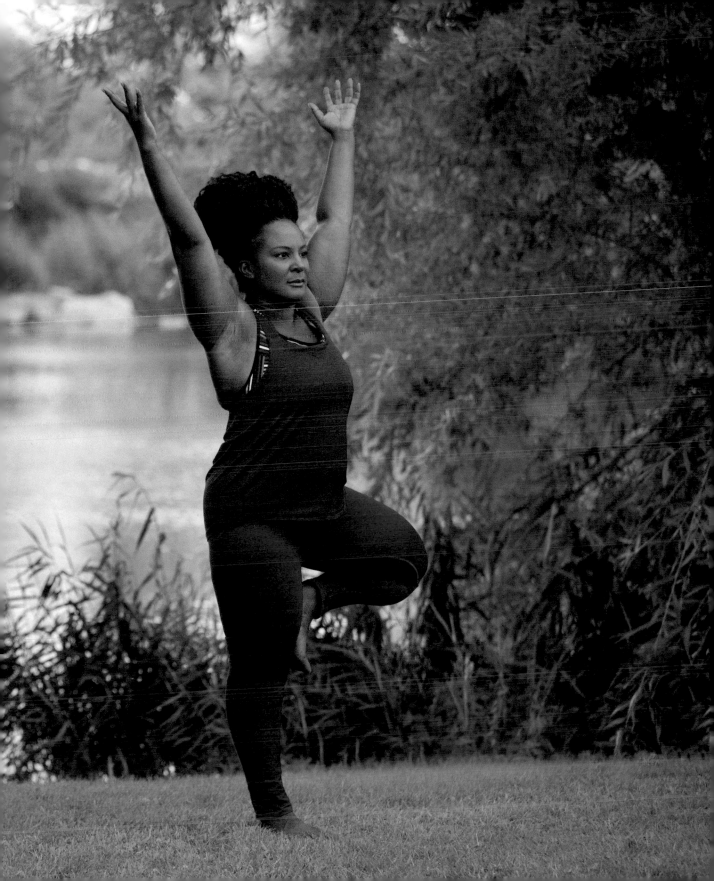

Happy Baby

>>> ANANDA BALASANA <<<

This pose might have a fun name, but don't let that fool you into thinking it's easy. This popular hip opener can help with mobility and tight muscles. You'll especially stretch the muscles of your inner thighs, groin, and lower back.

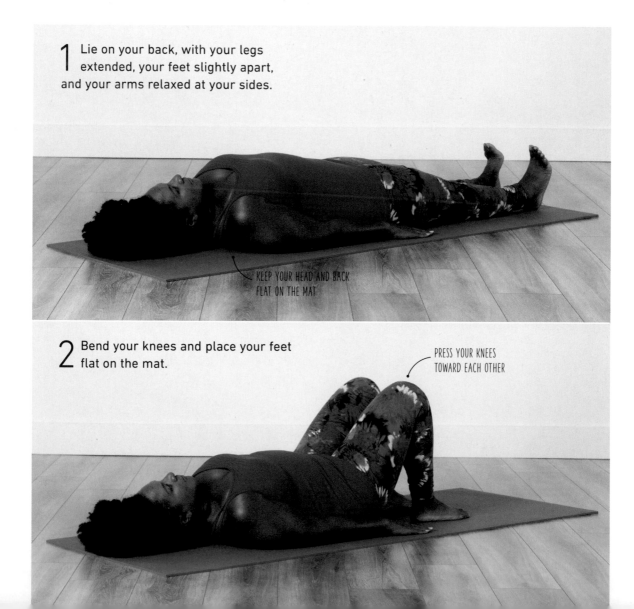

1 Lie on your back, with your legs extended, your feet slightly apart, and your arms relaxed at your sides.

KEEP YOUR HEAD AND BACK FLAT ON THE MAT

2 Bend your knees and place your feet flat on the mat.

PRESS YOUR KNEES TOWARD EACH OTHER

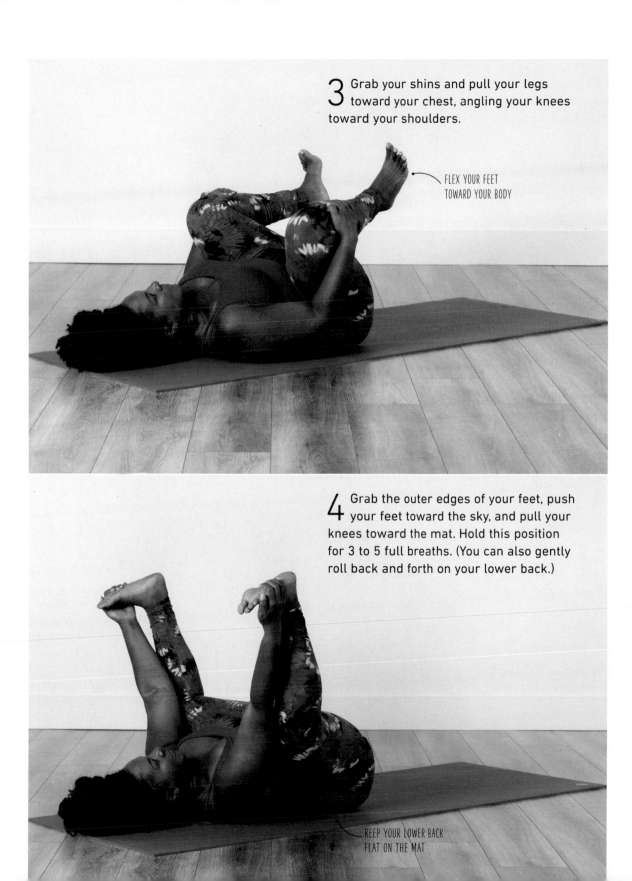

3 Grab your shins and pull your legs toward your chest, angling your knees toward your shoulders.

FLEX YOUR FEET
TOWARD YOUR BODY

4 Grab the outer edges of your feet, push your feet toward the sky, and pull your knees toward the mat. Hold this position for 3 to 5 full breaths. (You can also gently roll back and forth on your lower back.)

KEEP YOUR LOWER BACK
FLAT ON THE MAT

~ HAPPY BABY ~

VARIATIONS

Happy Baby can be a joyful pose, but if you have trouble getting into and maintaining this position, these variations can help you better enjoy this experience.

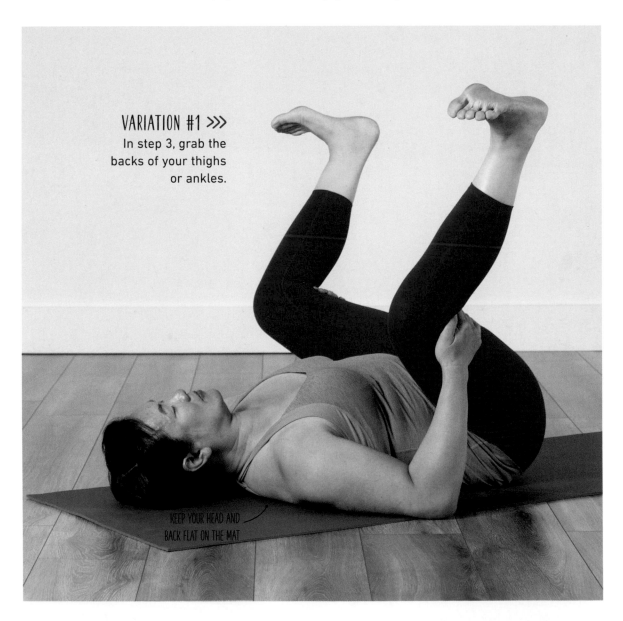

VARIATION #1 >>>
In step 3, grab the backs of your thighs or ankles.

KEEP YOUR HEAD AND BACK FLAT ON THE MAT

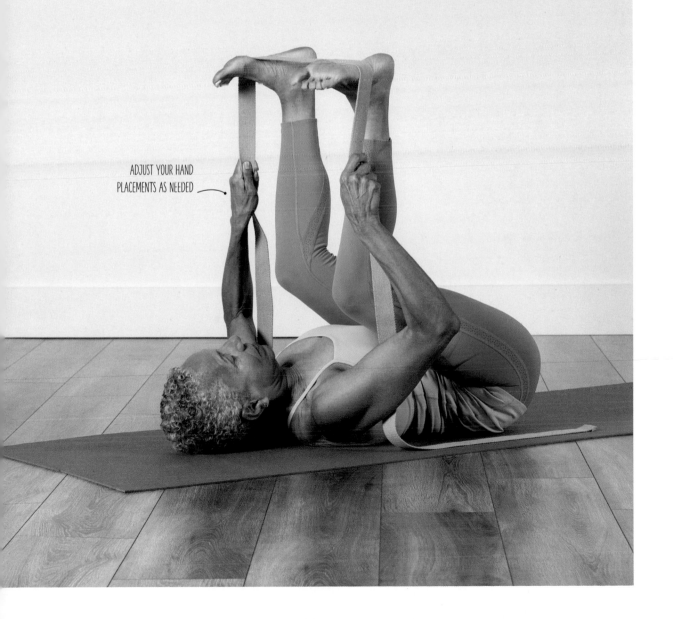

≪≪≪ VARIATION #2

Wrap a strap around your feet. In step 3, hold an end of the strap in each hand. In step 4, press your feet into the strap and widen your knees.

ADJUST YOUR HAND
PLACEMENTS AS NEEDED

Easy Pose

>>> SUKHASANA <<<

You might recognize this seated cross-legged pose as a classic position in yoga. Despite the name of this pose, your movements require focus and balance, which this pose can help you develop and strengthen.

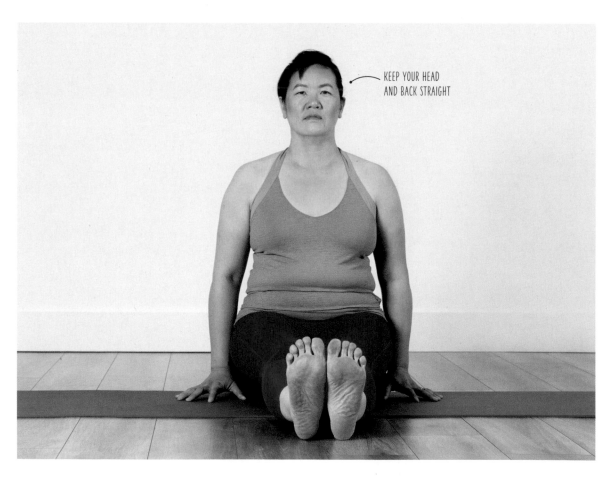

KEEP YOUR HEAD AND BACK STRAIGHT

1 Sit on a block, with your legs extended and your arms relaxed at your sides. Press your sitting bones into the mat for support and lengthen your spine through the crown of your head.

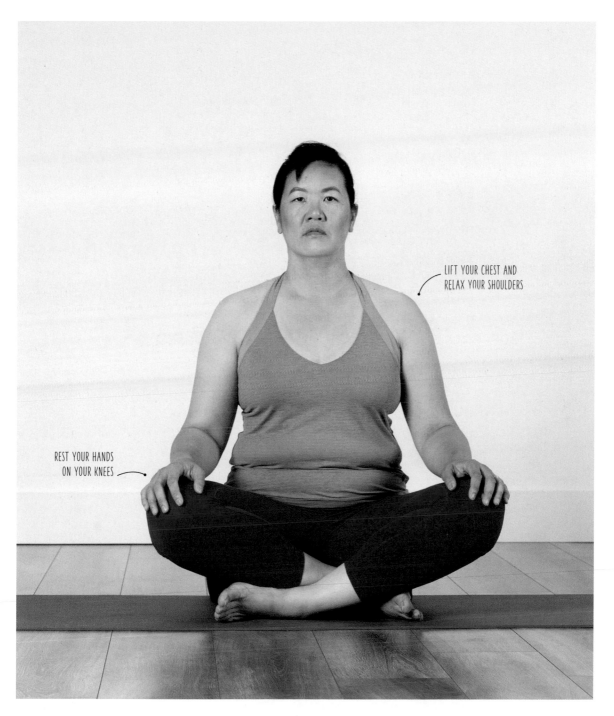

LIFT YOUR CHEST AND
RELAX YOUR SHOULDERS

REST YOUR HANDS
ON YOUR KNEES

2 Bend your right knee and bring your right heel as close to
your sitting bones as possible. Bend your left knee and
bring your left heel as close to your sitting bones as possible,
aligning the front of your right ankle with the back of your
left ankle. Hold this position for 3 to 5 full breaths.

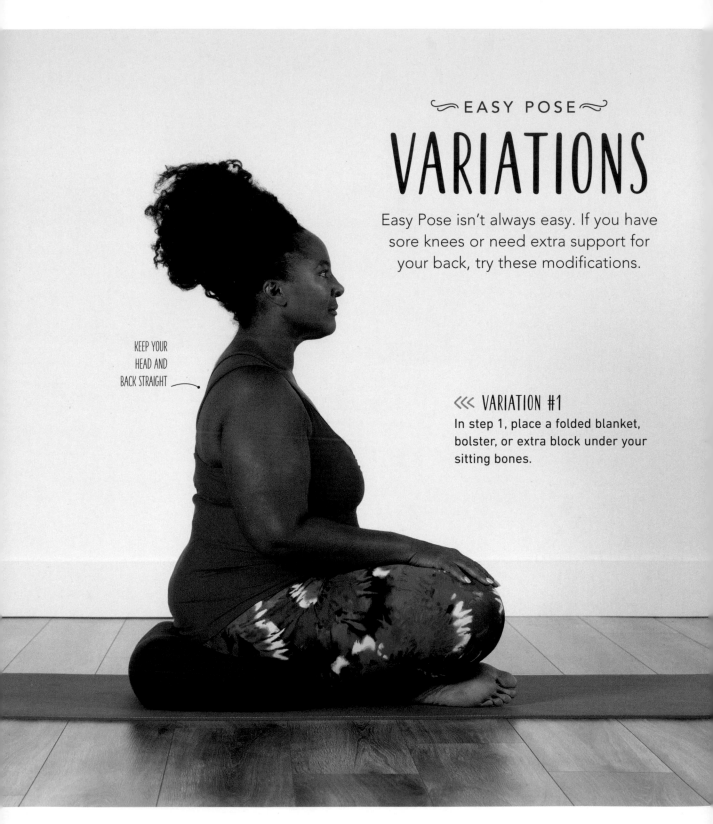

VARIATIONS

Easy Pose isn't always easy. If you have sore knees or need extra support for your back, try these modifications.

KEEP YOUR
HEAD AND
BACK STRAIGHT

⫷ VARIATION #1

In step 1, place a folded blanket, bolster, or extra block under your sitting bones.

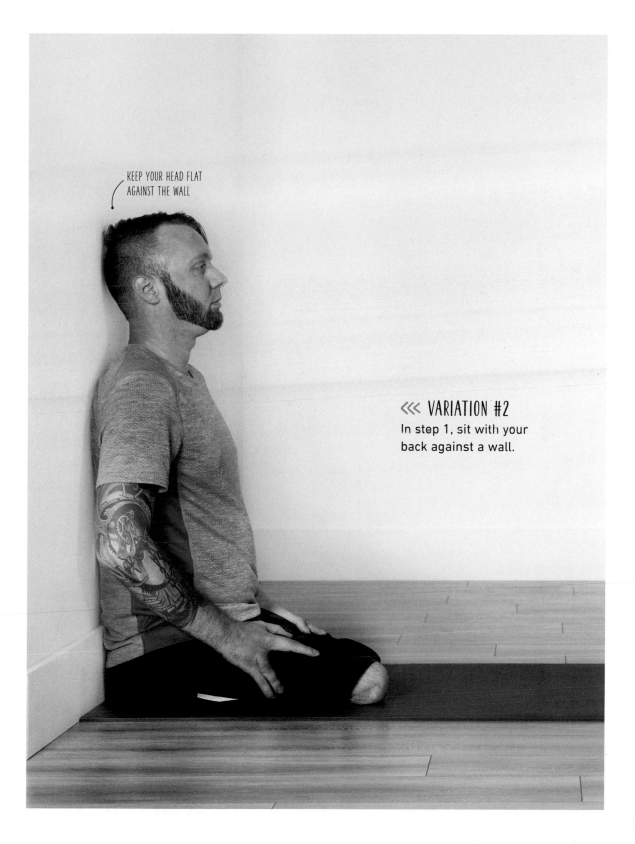

KEEP YOUR HEAD FLAT
AGAINST THE WALL

⟪ VARIATION #2

In step 1, sit with your
back against a wall.

Child's Pose

>>> SUPTA BALASANA <<<

Considered a resting pose, this is often known as the pose of surrender—but the good kind. You'll feel a stretch in your spine, shoulders, hips, and thighs. And have some fun during this pose to intensify the results.

1 Place your hands, knees, and the tops of your feet flat on the mat. Widen your knees as far apart as possible, with your lower legs angled inward until your big toes touch.

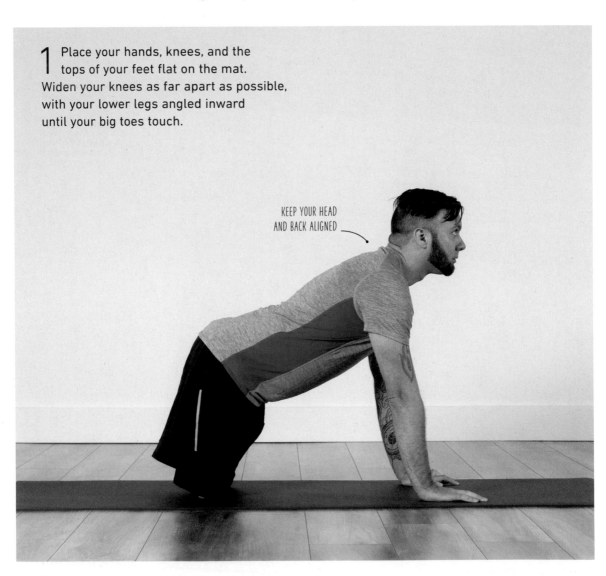

KEEP YOUR HEAD AND BACK ALIGNED

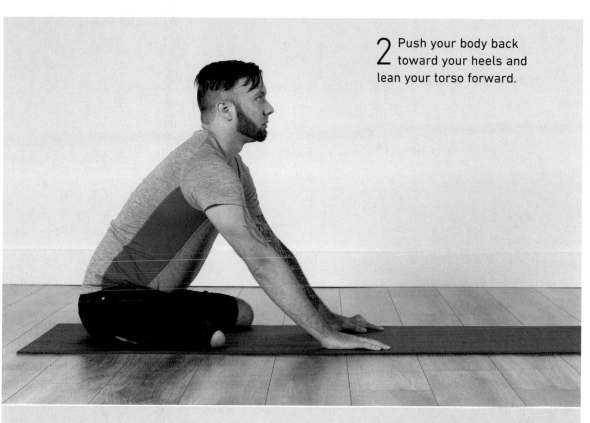

2 Push your body back toward your heels and lean your torso forward.

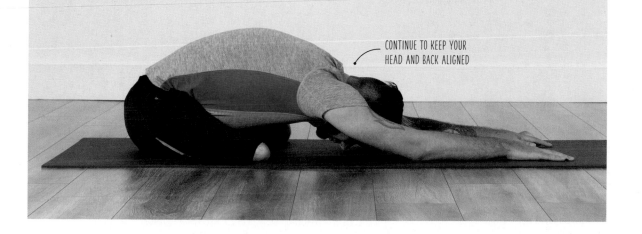

3 Extend your arms, slowly lowering your torso to the mat. Hold this position for 3 to 5 full breaths.

CONTINUE TO KEEP YOUR HEAD AND BACK ALIGNED

∽ CHILD'S POSE ∽
VARIATIONS

This pose is great for when you need an extra moment to catch your breath during practice. However, it can be uncomfortable for people with larger bodies or for anyone with previous or current knee injuries.

⟪ VARIATION #1

Place a rolled blanket or a small bolster nearby and a large bolster under your torso. In step 1, place the blanket or bolster behind your thighs and on top of your calves. In step 3, lower your torso onto the bolster and relax your arms at your sides.

ALLOW YOUR BACK
TO GENTLY CURVE
TOWARD YOUR HEAD

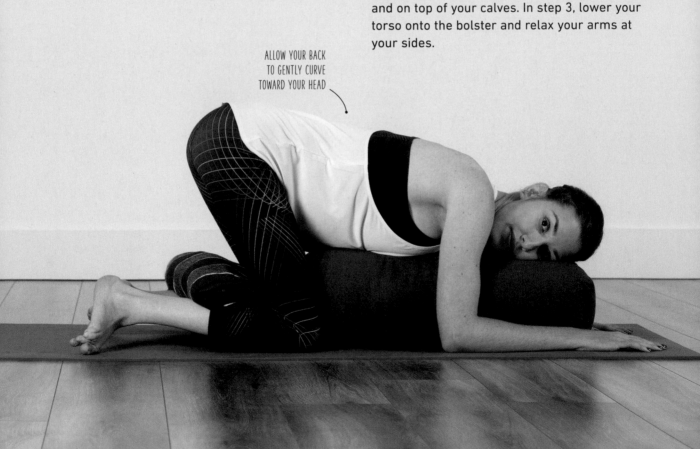

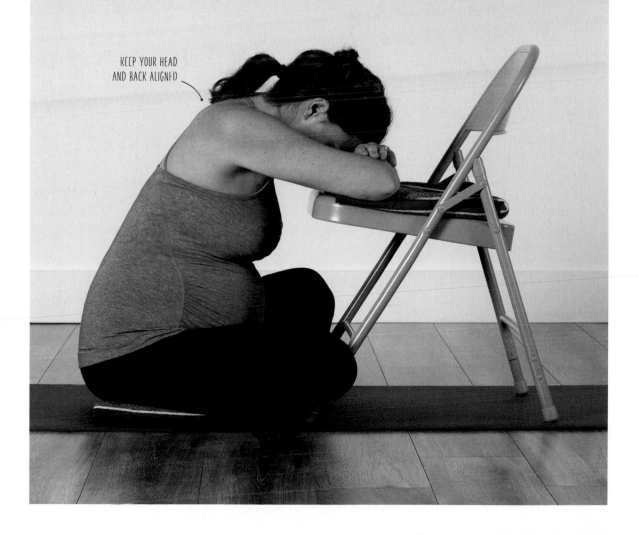

≪≪ VARIATION #2

1. Sit cross-legged (or place the soles of your feet together) on a rolled blanket or a small bolster and face the seat of a chair.
2. Lean your torso toward the seat of the chair, stack your forearms on the seat, and rest your head on your forearms. Hold this position for 3 to 5 full breaths.

KEEP YOUR HEAD AND BACK ALIGNED

Plank

>>>PHALAKASANA<<<

Performing this foundational yoga pose builds strength
in your shoulders, arms, and chest. In fact, this pose is one
of the fastest ways to develop better strength, and it's often
used for transitioning from pose to pose during a sequence.

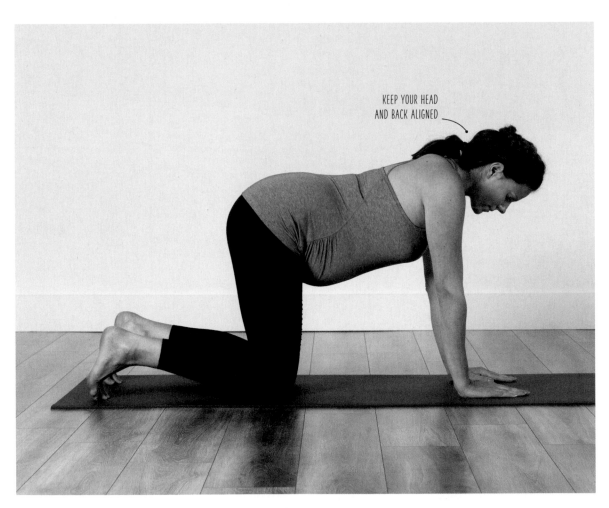

KEEP YOUR HEAD
AND BACK ALIGNED

1 Place your hands and knees flat on the mat,
with your toes curled under and your wrists
aligned with your shoulders.

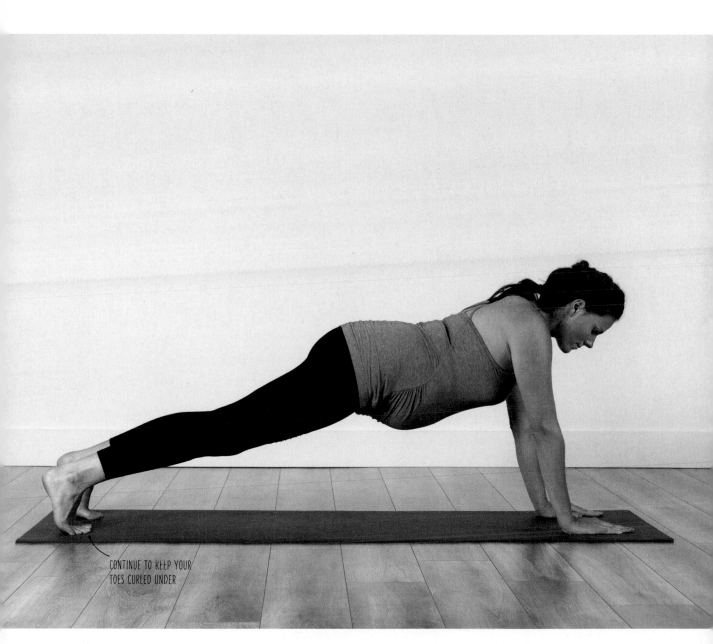

CONTINUE TO KEEP YOUR
TOES CURLED UNDER

2 Lift your knees off the ground until your legs are straight.
Press your hands into the mat to keep your body lifted.
Hold this position for 3 to 5 full breaths.

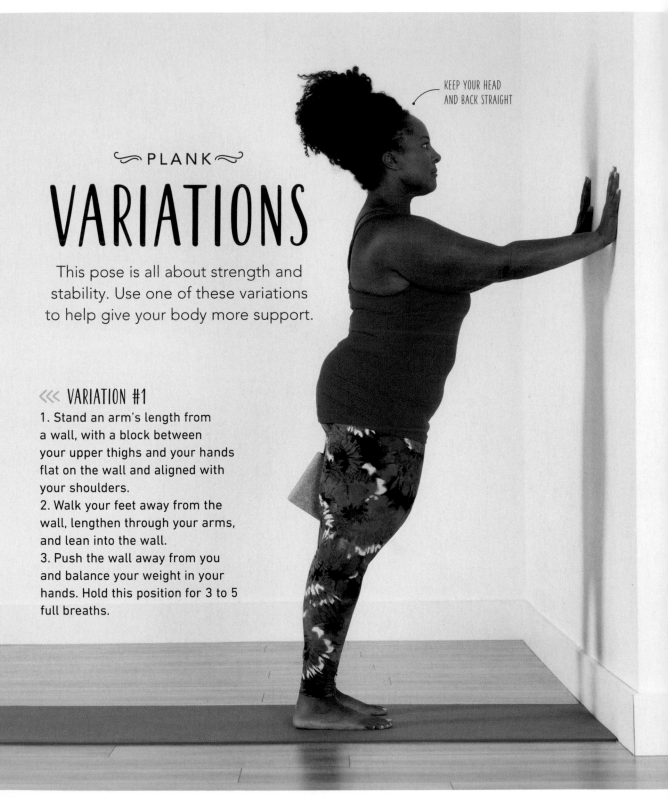

KEEP YOUR HEAD
AND BACK STRAIGHT

∼ PLANK ∼

VARIATIONS

This pose is all about strength and
stability. Use one of these variations
to help give your body more support.

‹‹‹ VARIATION #1

1. Stand an arm's length from
a wall, with a block between
your upper thighs and your hands
flat on the wall and aligned with
your shoulders.

2. Walk your feet away from the
wall, lengthen through your arms,
and lean into the wall.

3. Push the wall away from you
and balance your weight in your
hands. Hold this position for 3 to 5
full breaths.

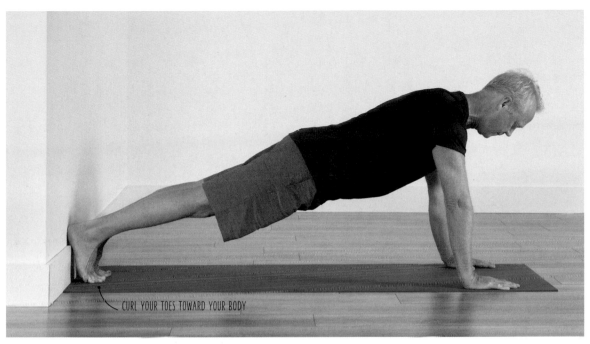

CURL YOUR TOES TOWARD YOUR BODY

⋘ VARIATION #2

Face away from a wall. In step 2, place your heels against the wall.

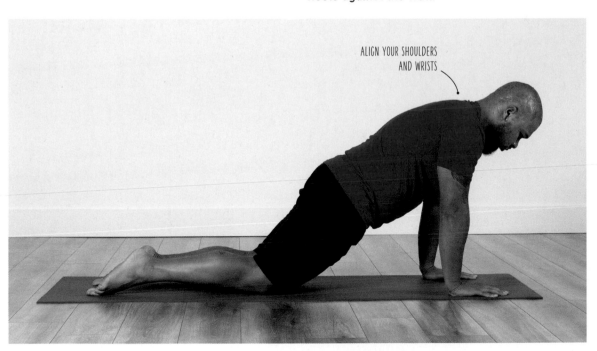

ALIGN YOUR SHOULDERS AND WRISTS

⋘ VARIATION #3

In step 2, keep your knees on the mat.

Low Plank

>>>CHATURANGA DANDASANA<<<

Although you might find this to be a physically challenging pose, just keep telling yourself that it can strengthen your upper-body stamina. To execute this pose, you must recruit your arms, shoulders, chest, and core muscles.

1 Place your hands and knees flat on the mat, with your toes curled under and your wrists and shoulders aligned.

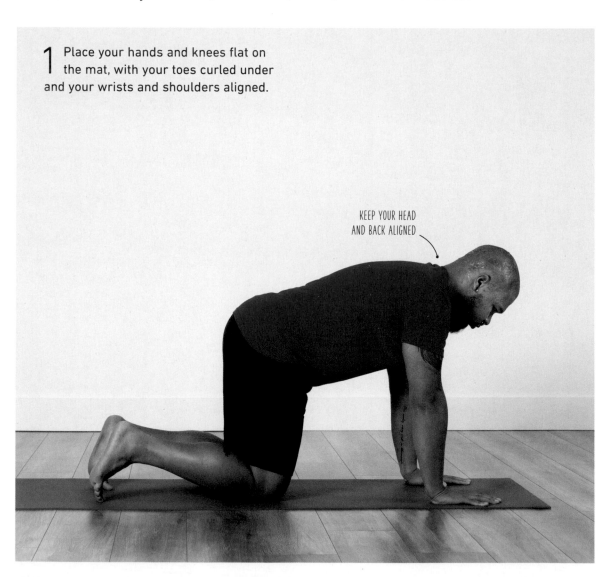

KEEP YOUR HEAD
AND BACK ALIGNED

2 Extend your legs behind you one at a time until your legs are straight, keeping your toes curled. Press your hands into the mat and push your heels away from your body.

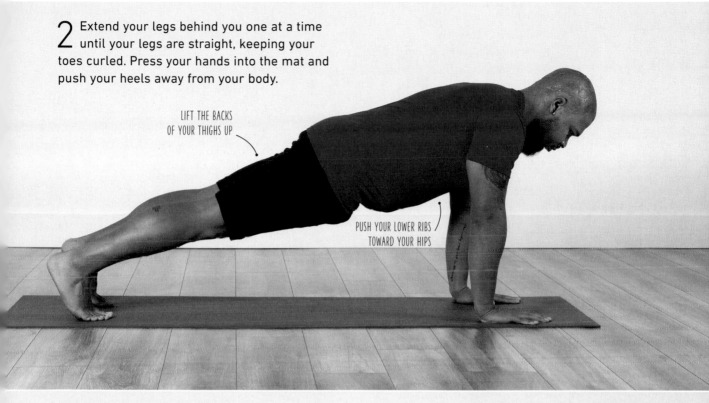

LIFT THE BACKS
OF YOUR THIGHS UP

PUSH YOUR LOWER RIBS
TOWARD YOUR HIPS

3 Bend your elbows and lower your body until your upper arms align with your torso, pulling your elbows toward your body and squeezing your thighs together. Hold this position for 3 to 5 full breaths.

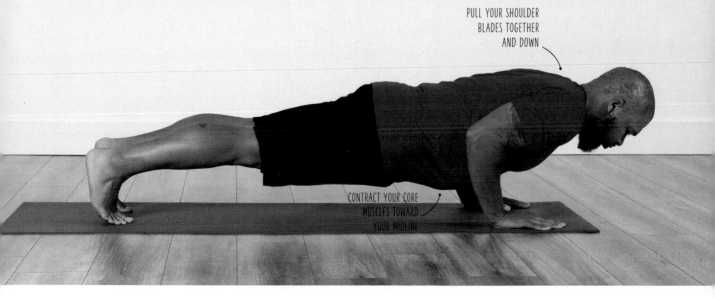

PULL YOUR SHOULDER
BLADES TOGETHER
AND DOWN

CONTRACT YOUR CORE
MUSCLES TOWARD
YOUR MIDLINE

~ LOW PLANK ~

VARIATIONS

This pose can be one of the toughest and most repetitive poses in yoga practice. Here are some ways to make this pose more accessible and to still build strength.

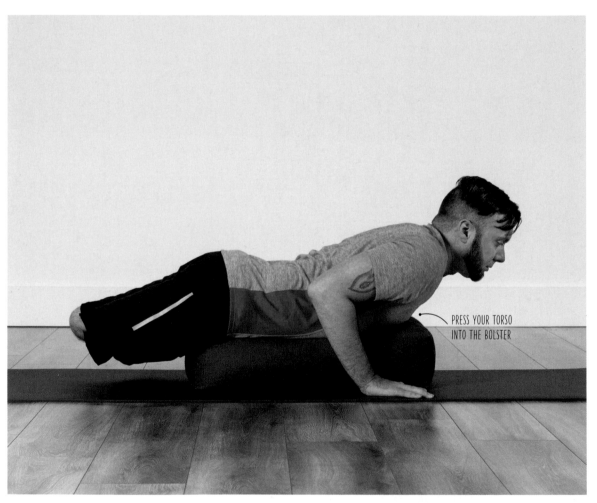

PRESS YOUR TORSO
INTO THE BOLSTER

⋘ VARIATION #1

Place a large bolster under your torso. In step 3, lower your body onto the bolster.

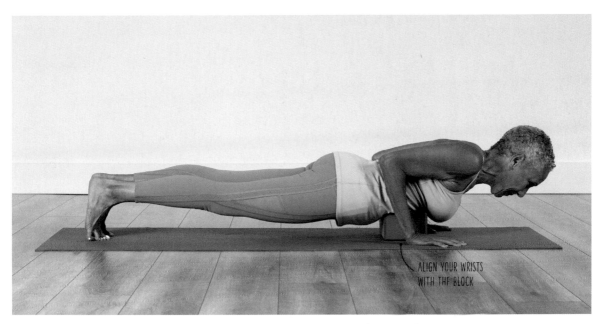

ALIGN YOUR WRISTS
WITH THE BLOCK

⟪ VARIATION #2

Place a block long side up on the mat under your torso. In step 3, lower your torso onto the block. (You can also perform this step with the block on its long edge.)

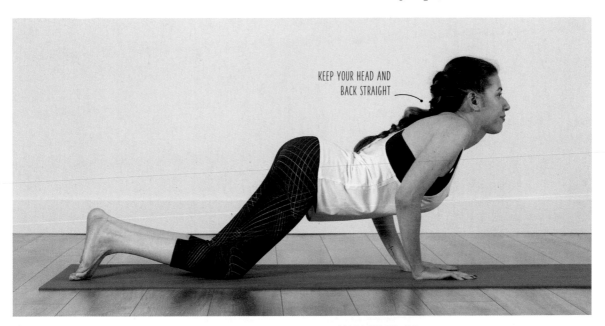

KEEP YOUR HEAD AND
BACK STRAIGHT

⟪ VARIATION #3

In step 2, keep one or both knees on the mat to support your weight.

Low Lunge

>>>ANJANEYASANA<<<

Sometimes known as Runner's Lunge, this pose stretches your quads, hamstrings, groin, and hips. This can also create more flexibility in your lower body, and it's great for anyone who needs some extra strength in their lower body.

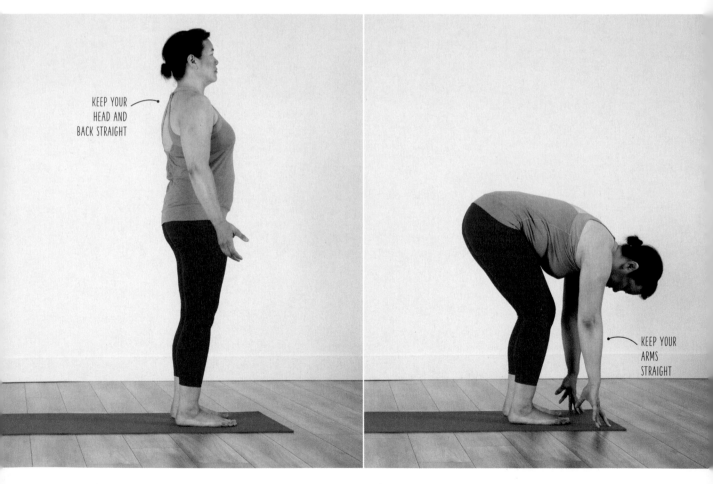

KEEP YOUR HEAD AND BACK STRAIGHT

KEEP YOUR ARMS STRAIGHT

1 Stand with your weight equally balanced between your feet and your arms relaxed at your sides.

2 Bend at your waist, lean your torso toward your thighs, and place your hands on the mat in front of you, slightly bending your knees.

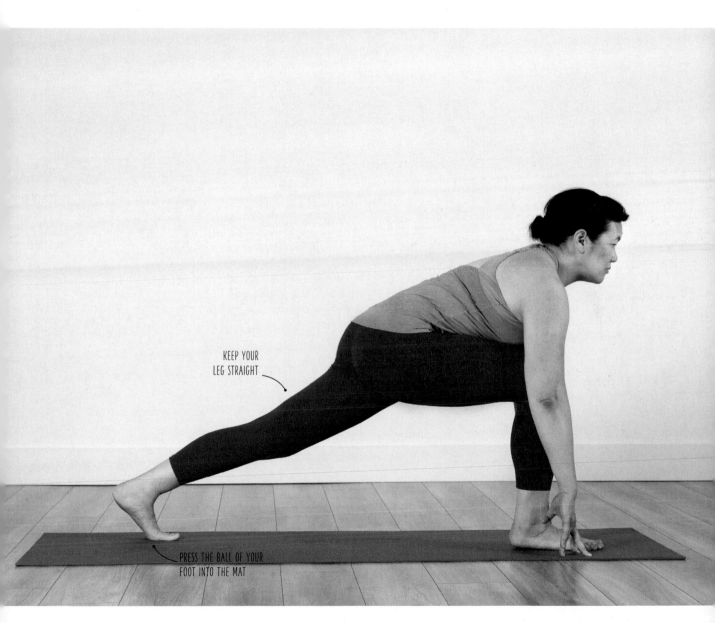

KEEP YOUR
LEG STRAIGHT

PRESS THE BALL OF YOUR
FOOT INTO THE MAT

3 Extend your left leg behind you and align your right knee
with your right ankle, lengthening your spine through the
crown of your head and looking forward. Hold this position
for 3 to 5 full breaths. Repeat these steps on the other side.

∽ LOW LUNGE ∽
VARIATIONS

If you find this pose too hard to get into or maintain, use some props to make it easier and more accessible.

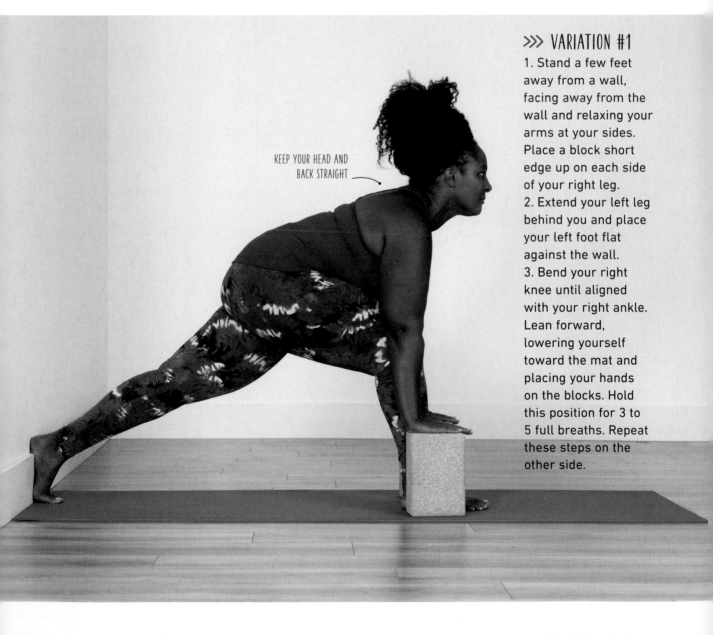

KEEP YOUR HEAD AND BACK STRAIGHT

>>> VARIATION #1

1. Stand a few feet away from a wall, facing away from the wall and relaxing your arms at your sides. Place a block short edge up on each side of your right leg.
2. Extend your left leg behind you and place your left foot flat against the wall.
3. Bend your right knee until aligned with your right ankle. Lean forward, lowering yourself toward the mat and placing your hands on the blocks. Hold this position for 3 to 5 full breaths. Repeat these steps on the other side.

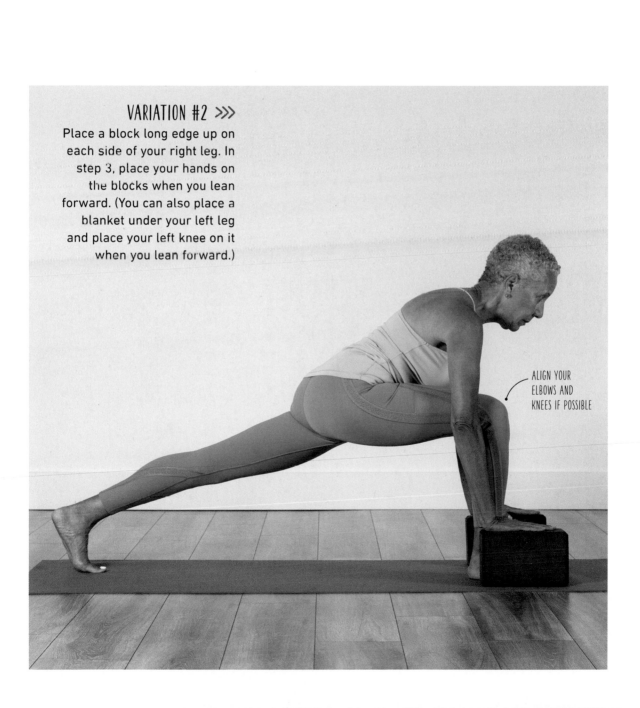

VARIATION #2 >>>

Place a block long edge up on each side of your right leg. In step 3, place your hands on the blocks when you lean forward. (You can also place a blanket under your left leg and place your left knee on it when you lean forward.)

ALIGN YOUR ELBOWS AND KNEES IF POSSIBLE

Extended Hand to Big Toe

>>>UTTHITA HASTA PADANGUSTHASANA<<<

This pose tests your balance and core strength while requiring an intense focus to help you hold the final position. These movements demand hamstring and hip flexibility, which this pose can also help you develop.

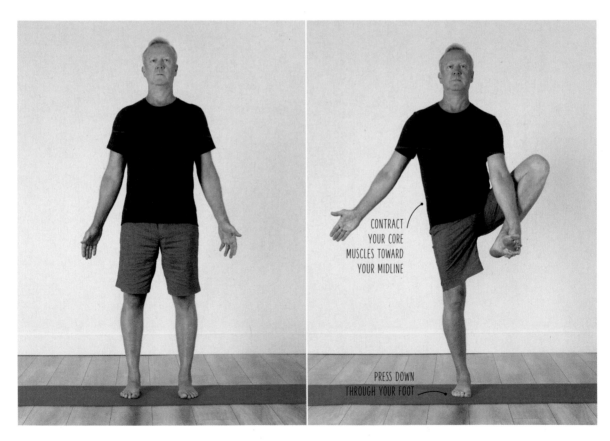

CONTRACT YOUR CORE MUSCLES TOWARD YOUR MIDLINE

PRESS DOWN THROUGH YOUR FOOT

1 Stand with your weight balanced equally between your feet and your arms relaxed at your sides.

2 Shift your weight to your right foot, bend your left knee, lift your left knee toward your left armpit, and wrap your left hand around the outer edge of your left foot.

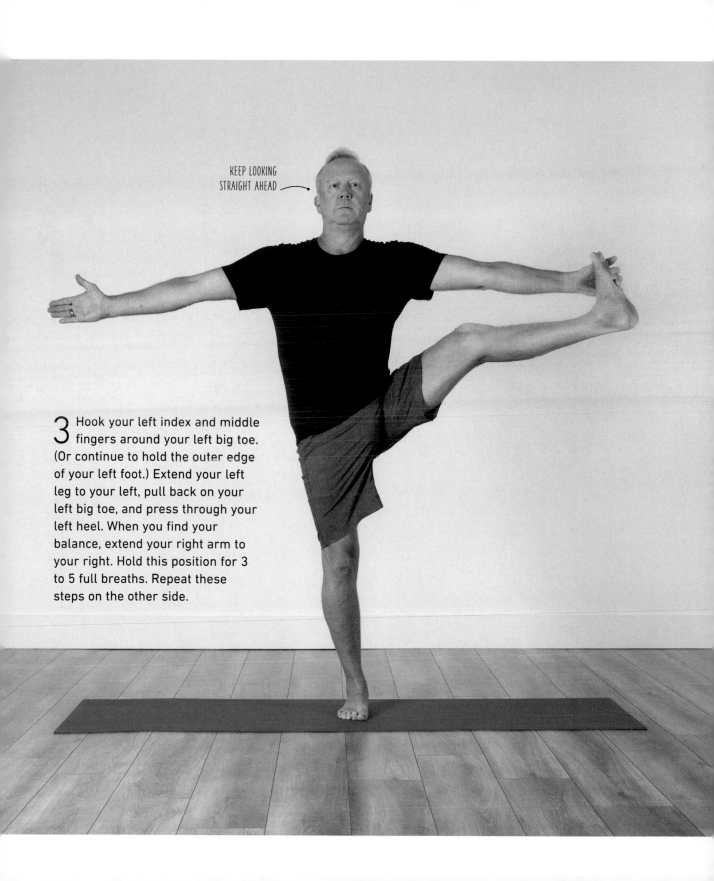

KEEP LOOKING STRAIGHT AHEAD

3 Hook your left index and middle fingers around your left big toe. (Or continue to hold the outer edge of your left foot.) Extend your left leg to your left, pull back on your left big toe, and press through your left heel. When you find your balance, extend your right arm to your right. Hold this position for 3 to 5 full breaths. Repeat these steps on the other side.

~ EXTENDED HAND TO BIG TOE ~
VARIATIONS

Using a strap, a wall, or a chair can help make this pose
more accessible—and much more enjoyable.

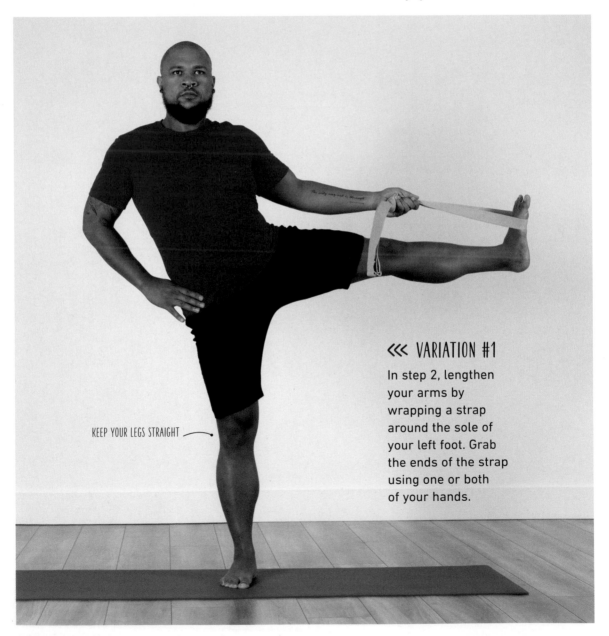

KEEP YOUR LEGS STRAIGHT

‹‹‹ VARIATION #1

In step 2, lengthen
your arms by
wrapping a strap
around the sole of
your left foot. Grab
the ends of the strap
using one or both
of your hands.

VARIATION #2 >>>

Place the seat of a chair against a wall. In step 3, place your left leg across the back of the chair and reach for your toes with your left hand.

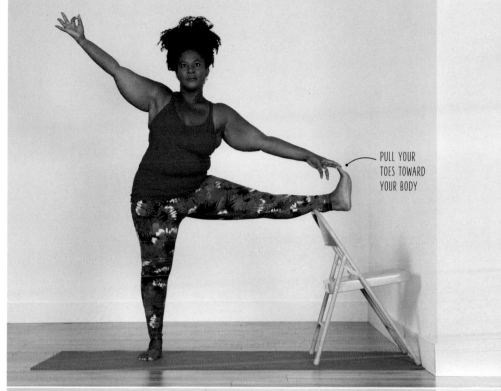

PULL YOUR TOES TOWARD YOUR BODY

VARIATION #3 >>>

In step 1, stand a leg's length away from a wall. In step 3, extend your left leg toward the wall and place your left foot flat against the wall.

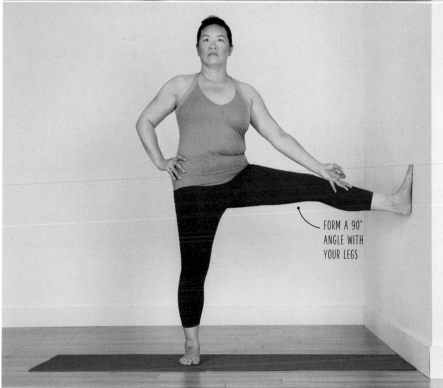

FORM A 90° ANGLE WITH YOUR LEGS

Reclining
Hand to Big Toe

>>>SUPTA PADANGUSTHASANA<<<

Are you looking for a way to give your hamstrings and lower back an incredible stretch? This pose can help you do that. The movements of this hip opener also stretch your hip flexors and your calf muscles.

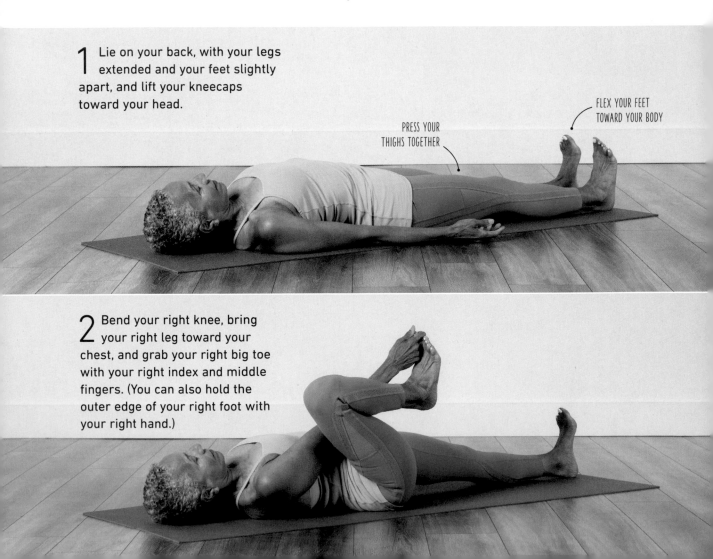

1 Lie on your back, with your legs extended and your feet slightly apart, and lift your kneecaps toward your head.

PRESS YOUR THIGHS TOGETHER

FLEX YOUR FEET TOWARD YOUR BODY

2 Bend your right knee, bring your right leg toward your chest, and grab your right big toe with your right index and middle fingers. (You can also hold the outer edge of your right foot with your right hand.)

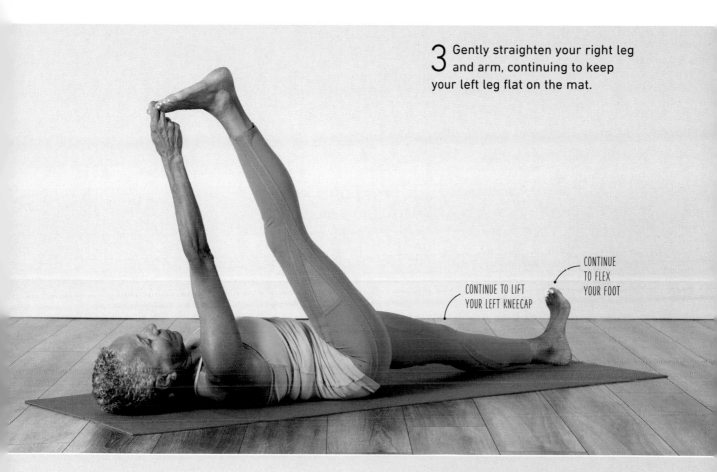

3 Gently straighten your right leg and arm, continuing to keep your left leg flat on the mat.

CONTINUE TO LIFT YOUR LEFT KNEECAP

CONTINUE TO FLEX YOUR FOOT

4 Extend your right leg to your right and extend your left arm to your left. Hold this position for 3 to 5 full breaths. Repeat these steps on the other side.

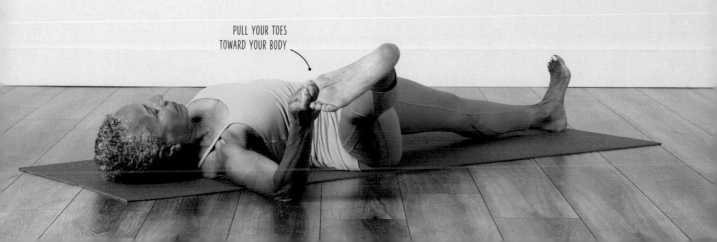

PULL YOUR TOES TOWARD YOUR BODY

~ RECLINING HAND TO BIG TOE ~
VARIATIONS

Most of us have legs that are longer than our arms.
This disproportionate ratio can make this pose challenging.
Fortunately, these variations can help this pose
feel more accessible.

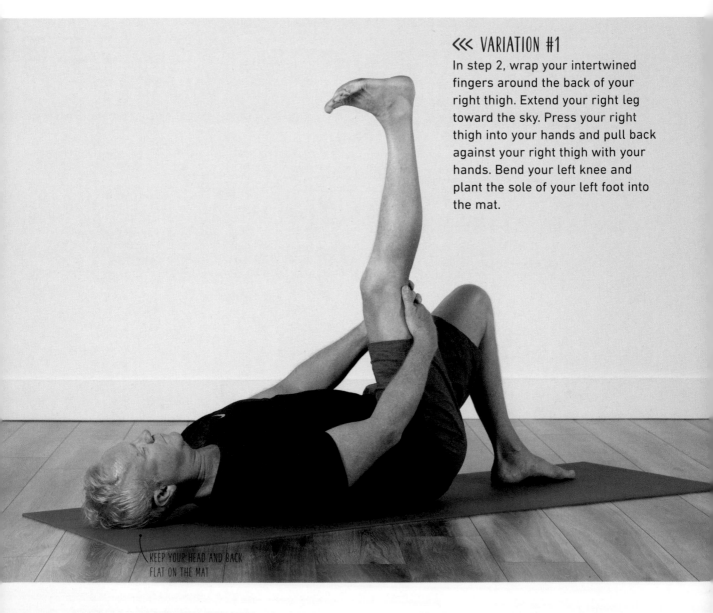

≪ VARIATION #1

In step 2, wrap your intertwined fingers around the back of your right thigh. Extend your right leg toward the sky. Press your right thigh into your hands and pull back against your right thigh with your hands. Bend your left knee and plant the sole of your left foot into the mat.

KEEP YOUR HEAD AND BACK
FLAT ON THE MAT

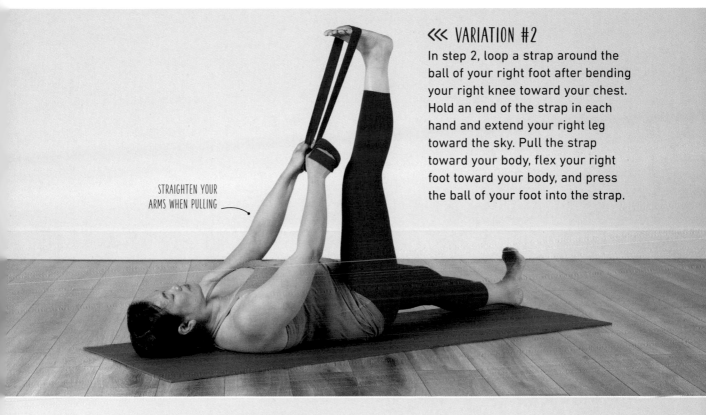

≪≪ VARIATION #2

In step 2, loop a strap around the ball of your right foot after bending your right knee toward your chest. Hold an end of the strap in each hand and extend your right leg toward the sky. Pull the strap toward your body, flex your right foot toward your body, and press the ball of your foot into the strap.

STRAIGHTEN YOUR
ARMS WHEN PULLING

VARIATION #3 ≫≫

Place a bolster or a block to the right of your right leg. In step 2, bend your right knee toward your chest and keep your left leg extended. In step 3, extend your right leg to your right and place it on the block or bolster. Extend your arms to form a T.

FLEX YOUR FEET
TOWARD YOUR BODY

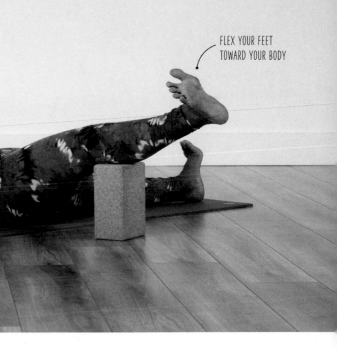

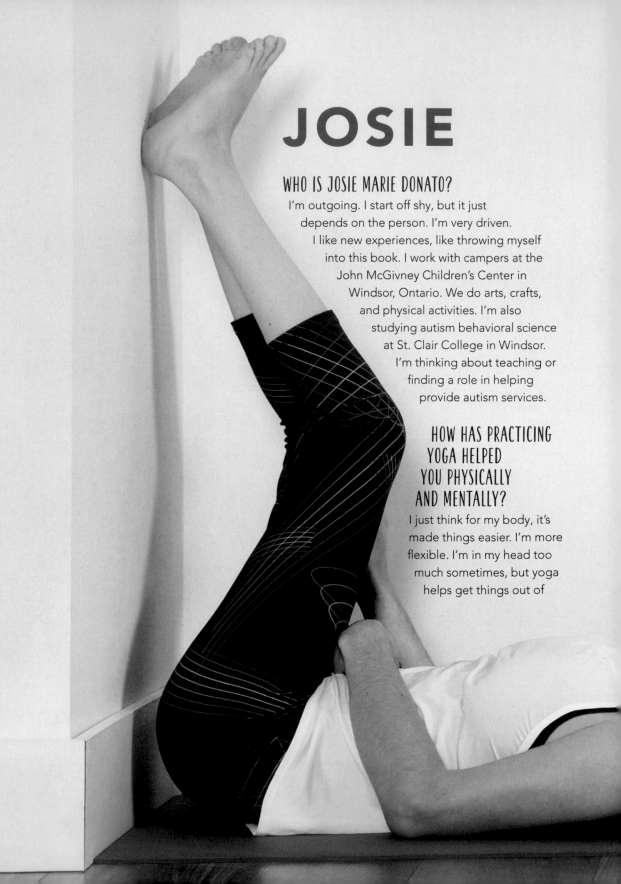

JOSIE

WHO IS JOSIE MARIE DONATO?

I'm outgoing. I start off shy, but it just depends on the person. I'm very driven. I like new experiences, like throwing myself into this book. I work with campers at the John McGivney Children's Center in Windsor, Ontario. We do arts, crafts, and physical activities. I'm also studying autism behavioral science at St. Clair College in Windsor. I'm thinking about teaching or finding a role in helping provide autism services.

HOW HAS PRACTICING YOGA HELPED YOU PHYSICALLY AND MENTALLY?

I just think for my body, it's made things easier. I'm more flexible. I'm in my head too much sometimes, but yoga helps get things out of my head. I just think about what I'm doing in that moment—and I stay very much in that moment. It's easier to do yoga than some other things because it's calm. Very peaceful. The expectations are there to know there's no chaos.

I'd like to get better. I'm comfortable doing most of the poses. I'm open to trying to do whatever's being asked of me. I'll get more comfortable and better with time. I want to see if I can hold a position longer each time I practice a pose.

I'm learning to be open to the experience. To be open to chanting and laughing. There are many parts of yoga that can be intimidating. I just have to get into others' ways of doing it. There's a tone. It's very encouraging. It helps with movements and positions. You have to breathe through it—even if it hurts. Center your breathing even when the breathing is difficult.

WHAT ARE YOUR GOALS WITH YOGA?

Putting myself out there even though I practice privately—just the yoga teacher and me right now. I'm getting used to being in front of other people. I don't want people to see me contorting to try to get into a pose. But after my first time practicing, no one was judgmental. I felt good. I felt instant comfort.

I'm becoming more comfortable with my instructor. My goal is to do these things on my own and have the confidence to do them. It's not as intimidating as it seems. I just need to keep trying to put myself out there. My instructor modifies poses to my ability and I don't worry about how it looks.

It's intimidating to be inspirational to others with cerebral palsy or other kinds of physical challenges. I feel better, though, after I push myself through something difficult and find success. I love the challenges that yoga encourages me to overcome. Building confidence is good.

FAVORITE POSE
>>> LEGS UP THE WALL

MOST CHALLENGING POSE
>>> LOW LUNGE

OCCUPATION
>>> CAMP COUNSELOR FOR KIDS WITH DISABILITIES

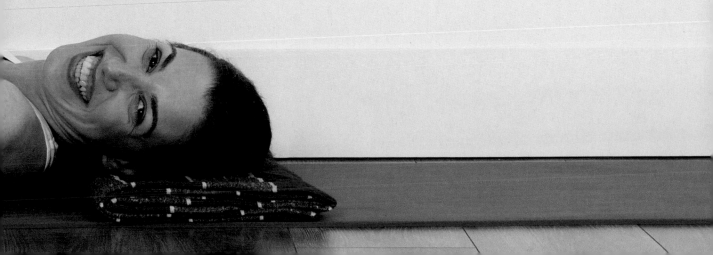

Handstand

>>>ADHO MUKHA VRKSASANA<<<

This challenging pose requires a great deal of upper-body strength, especially from your arms, chest, and upper back. It also demands balance, focus, determination, and practice, making this pose exhilarating and terrifying.

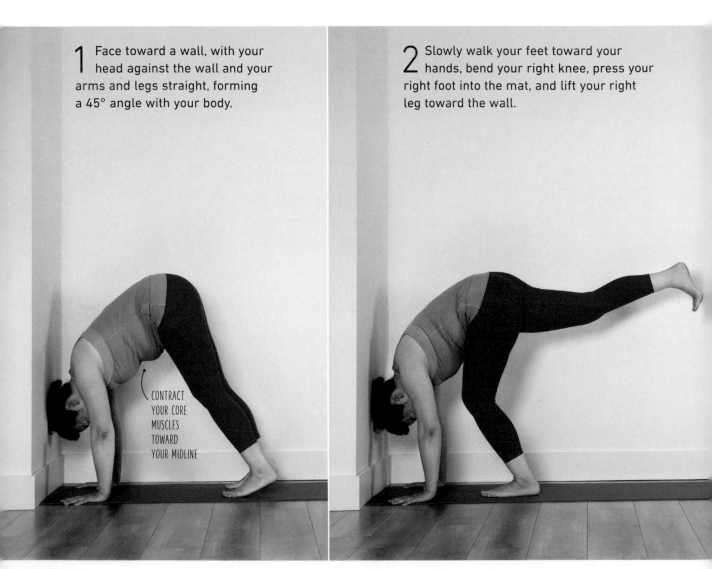

1 Face toward a wall, with your head against the wall and your arms and legs straight, forming a 45° angle with your body.

CONTRACT YOUR CORE MUSCLES TOWARD YOUR MIDLINE

2 Slowly walk your feet toward your hands, bend your right knee, press your right foot into the mat, and lift your right leg toward the wall.

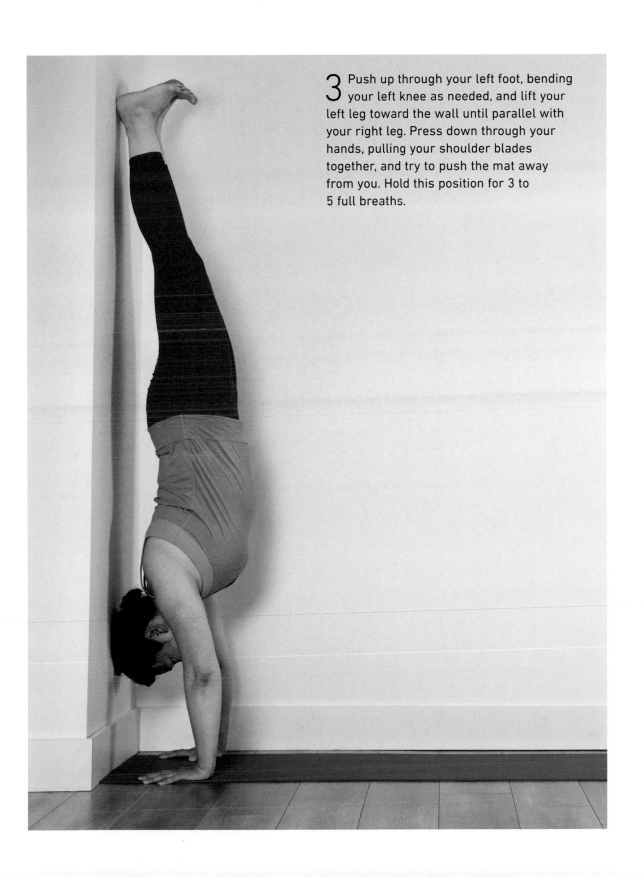

3 Push up through your left foot, bending your left knee as needed, and lift your left leg toward the wall until parallel with your right leg. Press down through your hands, pulling your shoulder blades together, and try to push the mat away from you. Hold this position for 3 to 5 full breaths.

⌒ HANDSTAND ⌒
VARIATIONS

Handstands help create strength and alleviate fear, but they aren't easy. These variations give you similar benefits to the main handstand—but in a more accessible way.

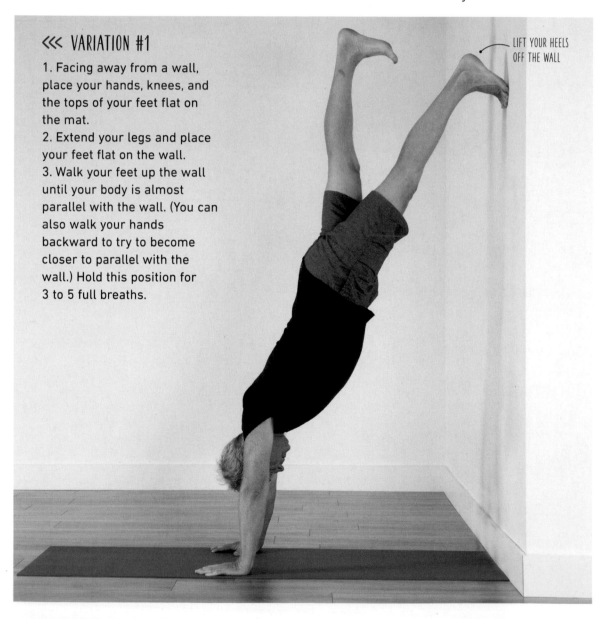

⋘ VARIATION #1

1. Facing away from a wall, place your hands, knees, and the tops of your feet flat on the mat.
2. Extend your legs and place your feet flat on the wall.
3. Walk your feet up the wall until your body is almost parallel with the wall. (You can also walk your hands backward to try to become closer to parallel with the wall.) Hold this position for 3 to 5 full breaths.

LIFT YOUR HEELS OFF THE WALL

««« VARIATION #2

1. Facing away from a wall, place your hands and knees flat on the mat and place your feet flat against the base of the wall.

2. Lift your knees off the mat and walk your legs up the wall until they're parallel with the mat. Pull your shoulder blades together, keep your legs straight, and press down through your hands to push the mat away from you. (For an added benefit, extend either leg toward the sky. Hold this position for 3 to 5 full breaths. Return that leg to the wall and extend your other leg toward the sky.)

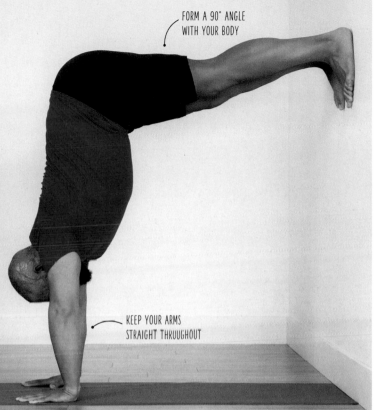

FORM A 90° ANGLE WITH YOUR BODY

KEEP YOUR ARMS STRAIGHT THROUGHOUT

««« VARIATION #3

1. Facing away from a wall, lie on your back, with your arms extended overhead, your fingertips touching the mat, and your feet pressed into the base of the wall.

2. Lift your kneecaps toward your head and flex your feet toward your body. Press down through your feet and press out through your hands. Hold this position for 3 to 5 full breaths.

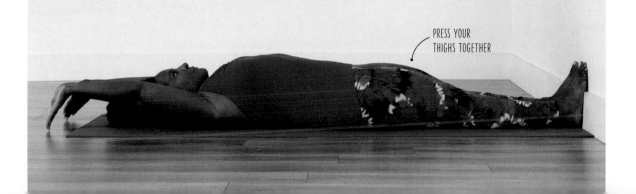

PRESS YOUR THIGHS TOGETHER

Forearm Stand

>>> PINCHA MAYURASANA <<<

This is an excellent pose for strengthening your arms, shoulders, upper back, and core muscles. These movements ask a lot of you—from strength and balance to focus and courage—but with continual practice, you can handle them.

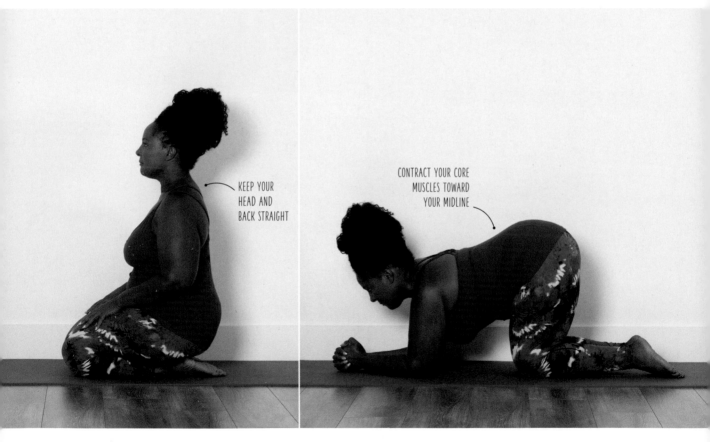

KEEP YOUR HEAD AND BACK STRAIGHT

CONTRACT YOUR CORE MUSCLES TOWARD YOUR MIDLINE

1 Facing a wall, kneel in the middle of the mat, with the tops of your feet flat on the mat and your hands resting on your thighs.

2 Intertwine your fingers and place your forearms flat on the mat, with your elbows aligned under your shoulders.

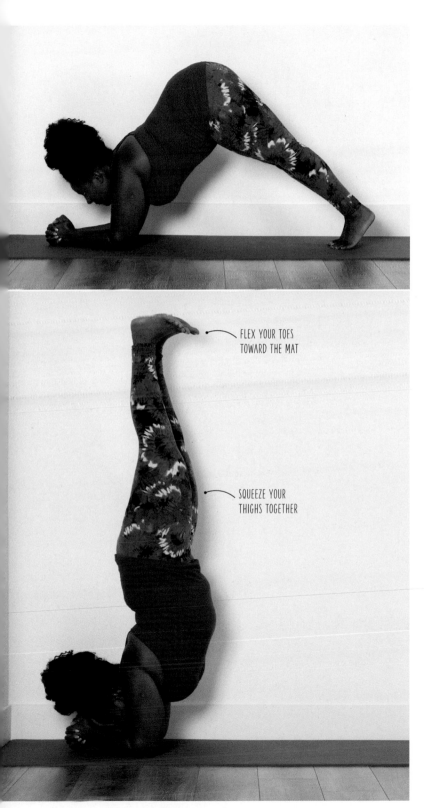

FLEX YOUR TOES
TOWARD THE MAT

SQUEEZE YOUR
THIGHS TOGETHER

3 Lift your knees off the mat and walk your feet toward your shoulders, pressing down through your forearms, pulling your shoulder blades together, and pressing your upper arms toward each other.

4 Lift your left leg toward the wall. Once you find your balance, lift your right leg until parallel with your left leg, using your forearms to help maintain your balance. Press your thighs together and push up through your heels. Hold this position for 3 to 5 full breaths.

∽ FOREARM STAND ∽
VARIATIONS

You can use different starting positions and a wall to help with these alternatives that come with similar benefits to the main pose but offer more support.

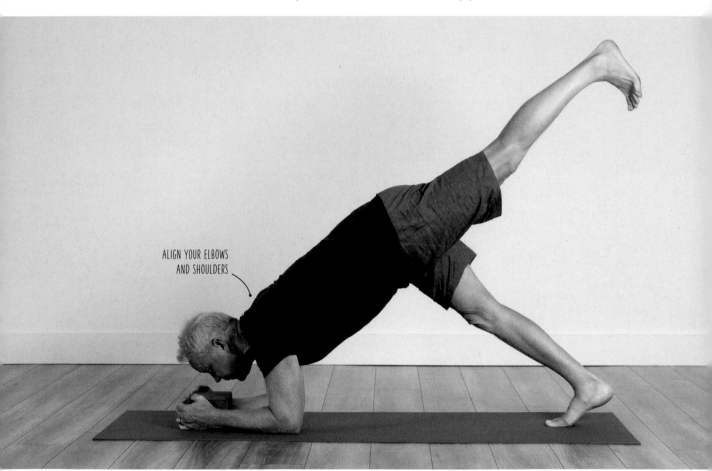

ALIGN YOUR ELBOWS AND SHOULDERS

⟪ VARIATION #1

In step 2, place a block long side up between your hands. In step 3, press your hands into the sides of the block. In step 4, extend your left leg until aligned with your torso. Hold this position for 3 to 5 full breaths. Repeat these steps on the other side.

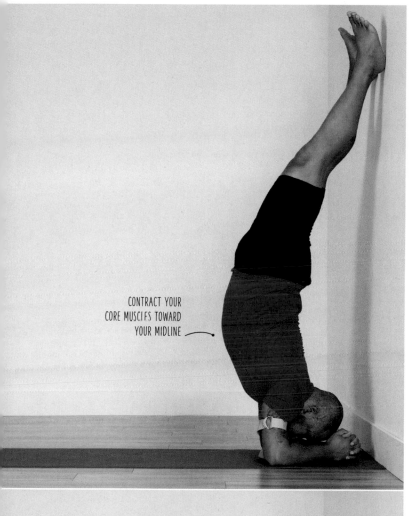

CONTRACT YOUR
CORE MUSCLES TOWARD
YOUR MIDLINE

‹‹‹ VARIATION #2

In step 1, face a wall and loop
a strap around your upper arms.
In step 4, lift your legs toward the
wall, resting your heels against the
wall and pressing down through
your forearms.

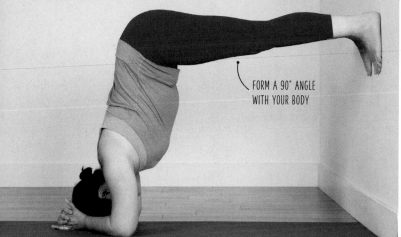

FORM A 90° ANGLE
WITH YOUR BODY

‹‹‹ VARIATION #3

1. Facing away from a wall, place
your knees flat on the mat, with
your feet flat against the base of
the wall and your hands interlaced
in front of you.
2. Walk your feet up the wall until
your legs are parallel with the mat.
Press down through your forearms
and pull your shoulder blades
together. Press your thighs
together and press the backs of
your legs toward the sky. Press
down through your forearms and
push the mat away from you. Hold
this position for 3 to 5 full breaths.

Wide-Angled
Seated Forward Fold

>>>UPAVISTHA KONASANA<<<

This is an excellent preparatory pose for deeper forward folds, twists, and wide-legged poses. These movements stretch your hamstrings, inner thighs, calves, glutes, and lower back, but your upper body won't be neglected.

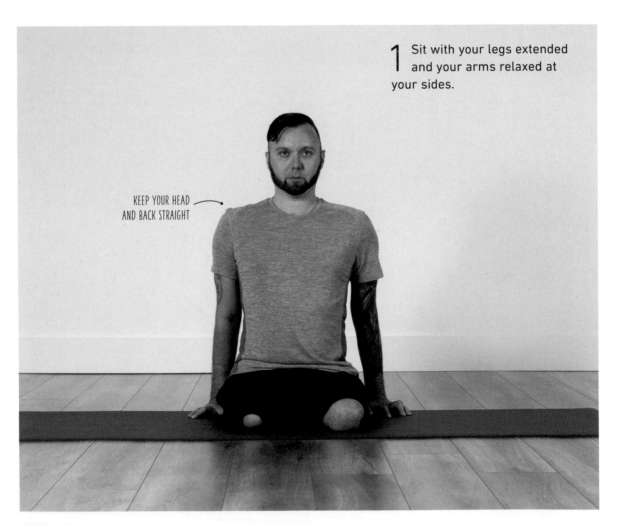

1 Sit with your legs extended and your arms relaxed at your sides.

KEEP YOUR HEAD AND BACK STRAIGHT

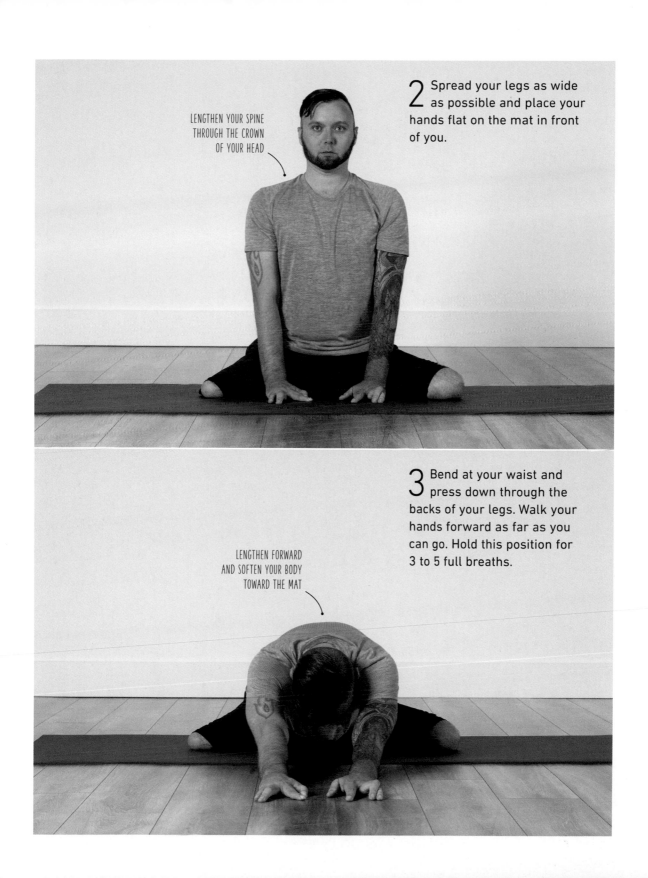

LENGTHEN YOUR SPINE
THROUGH THE CROWN
OF YOUR HEAD

2 Spread your legs as wide as possible and place your hands flat on the mat in front of you.

LENGTHEN FORWARD
AND SOFTEN YOUR BODY
TOWARD THE MAT

3 Bend at your waist and press down through the backs of your legs. Walk your hands forward as far as you can go. Hold this position for 3 to 5 full breaths.

⌣ WIDE-ANGLED SEATED FORWARD FOLD ⌣
VARIATIONS

Using a prop or wall can help alleviate stress on certain muscles as well as make this pose more accessible for a wide variety of body types.

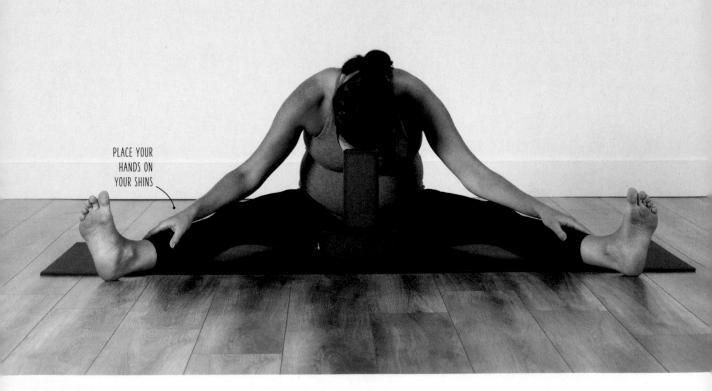

⟪ VARIATION #1

In step 2, place a block on the mat between your legs. (Add a second block as needed.) In step 3, touch your forehead to the block. (Adjust the placement of the block as needed as you lean forward. You can also place a rolled blanket under each knee.)

PLACE YOUR HANDS ON YOUR SHINS

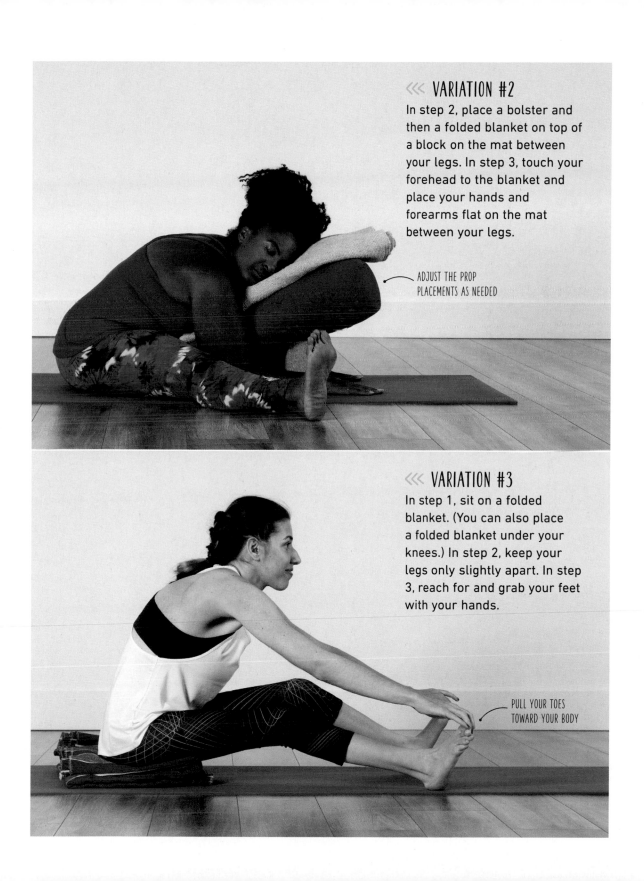

≪ VARIATION #2

In step 2, place a bolster and then a folded blanket on top of a block on the mat between your legs. In step 3, touch your forehead to the blanket and place your hands and forearms flat on the mat between your legs.

ADJUST THE PROP PLACEMENTS AS NEEDED

≪ VARIATION #3

In step 1, sit on a folded blanket. (You can also place a folded blanket under your knees.) In step 2, keep your legs only slightly apart. In step 3, reach for and grab your feet with your hands.

PULL YOUR TOES TOWARD YOUR BODY

Forward Fold

>>>UTTANASANA<<<

Helping you stretch your lower back, hamstrings, and calves, this pose offers grounding energy and can help recenter your thoughts. This pose's simple movements can also be a relaxing way to relieve stress in your body.

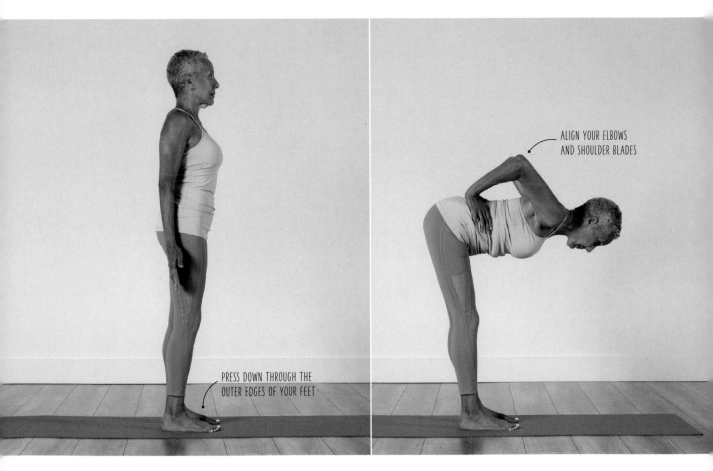

ALIGN YOUR ELBOWS AND SHOULDER BLADES

PRESS DOWN THROUGH THE OUTER EDGES OF YOUR FEET

1 Stand in the middle of the mat, with your weight balanced equally between your feet and your arms relaxed at your sides. Lift your toes off the mat, separate your toes, and anchor each toe into the mat.

2 Place your hands on your hips and gently bend at your waist, bringing your chest parallel with the mat and pulling your shoulder blades together. (Slightly bend your knees as needed for balance.)

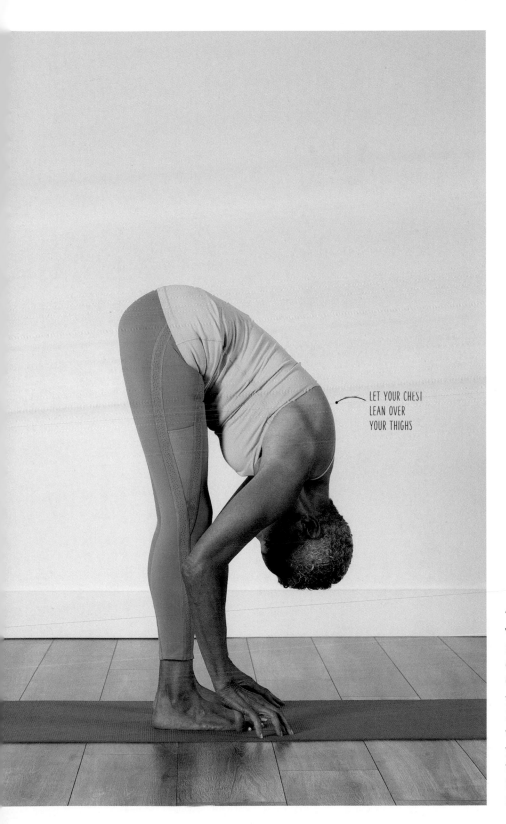

LET YOUR CHEST
LEAN OVER
YOUR THIGHS

3 Extend your arms
  toward the mat,
placing your fingertips
or hands on the mat.
(Or rest your hands on
your shins or feet.)
Push up through
where your legs meet
your buttocks—close
to your sitting bones.
Hold this position for
3 to 5 full breaths.

∽ FORWARD FOLD ∽
VARIATIONS

If you have tight hamstrings, a tight middle or lower back, or an abundance in the center of your body, this pose can prove difficult. But these variations can help.

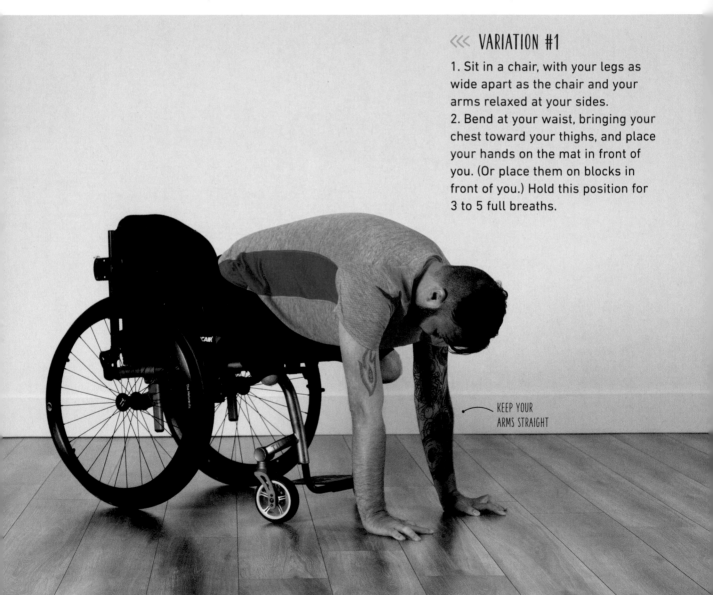

⋘ VARIATION #1

1. Sit in a chair, with your legs as wide apart as the chair and your arms relaxed at your sides.
2. Bend at your waist, bringing your chest toward your thighs, and place your hands on the mat in front of you. (Or place them on blocks in front of you.) Hold this position for 3 to 5 full breaths.

KEEP YOUR ARMS STRAIGHT

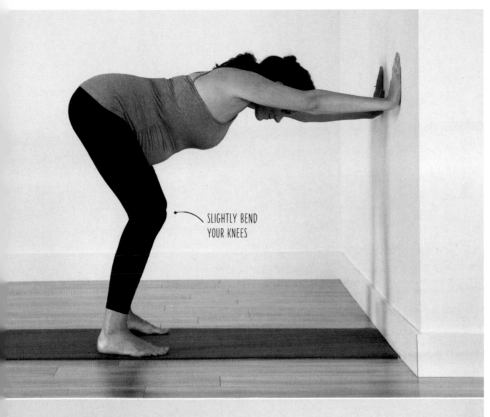

SLIGHTLY BEND YOUR KNEES

⫷ VARIATION #2

1. Facing an arm's distance away from a wall, place your hands flat on the wall. 2. Walk your feet backward and walk your hands down the wall until your torso is parallel with the mat. Hold this position for 3 to 5 full breaths.

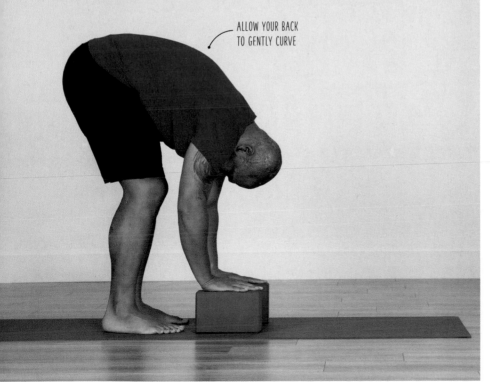

ALLOW YOUR BACK TO GENTLY CURVE

⫷ VARIATION #3

Place a block long edge up in front of each foot. In step 3, place your hands on the blocks when you bend and keep a slight bend in your knees. (Experiment with different heights by using more than one block per hand to help bring the mat closer to you.)

Head-to-Knee
Forward Fold

>>> JANU SIRSASANA <<<

Forward folds are essential components of a well-rounded
yoga practice because they're soothing and quieting for the
nervous system. Because this particular pose is one of the
more accessible forward folds, enjoy the calm it brings.

1 Sit on a folded blanket, with your legs
extended and your arms relaxed at your
sides. Lengthen your spine through the crown
of your head and press down through the backs
of your thighs.

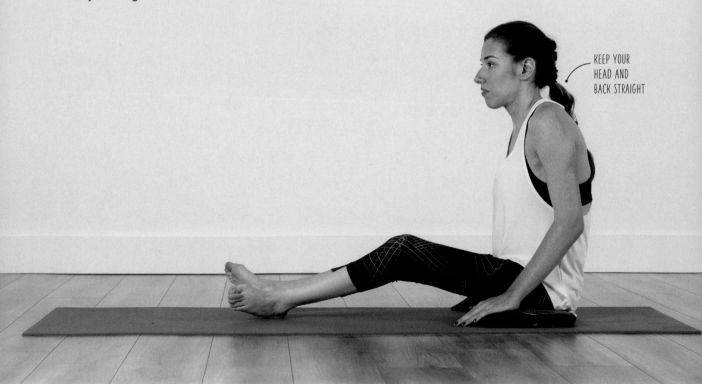

KEEP YOUR
HEAD AND
BACK STRAIGHT

2 Bend your left knee to bring the heel of your left foot toward your pubic bone, keeping your left foot flat on the mat. Press down through the back of your right leg. (Bend the knee of your extended right leg if you feel tightness in your hamstrings or lower back.)

PLACE YOUR HANDS
WHERE COMFORTABLE

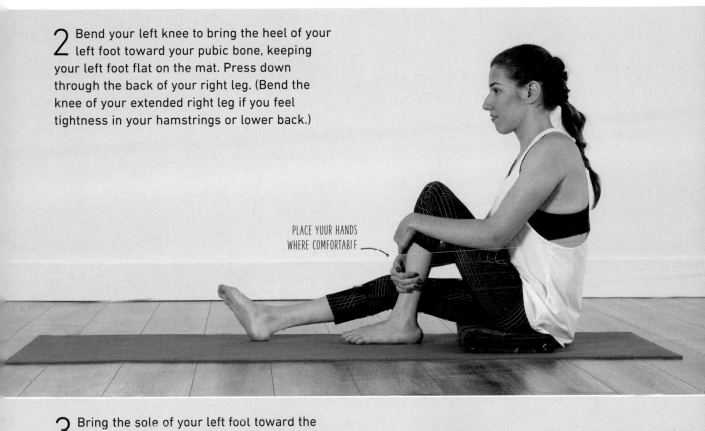

3 Bring the sole of your left foot toward the inside of your right leg. Align your body with your right leg and lengthen your spine toward your right foot. Walk your hands forward as far as you can and place your hands on your right shin. (You can also place your hands on the mat. If your left knee lifts too much, place a block under it for support.) Hold this position for 3 to 5 full breaths. Repeat these steps on the other side.

FLEX YOUR FOOT AWAY
FROM YOUR BODY

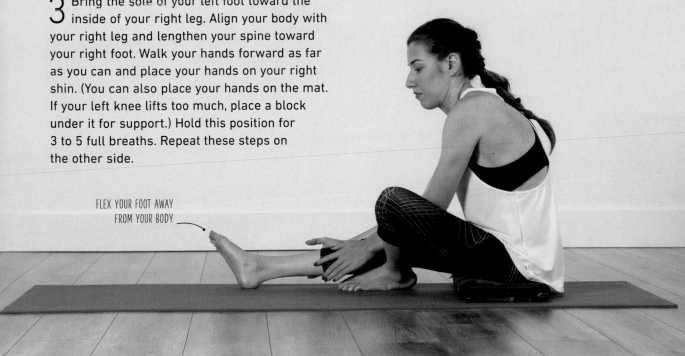

VARIATIONS

This is an excellent warmup or cooldown pose, and it has a few accessible variations that can help you enjoy all the benefits of these movements.

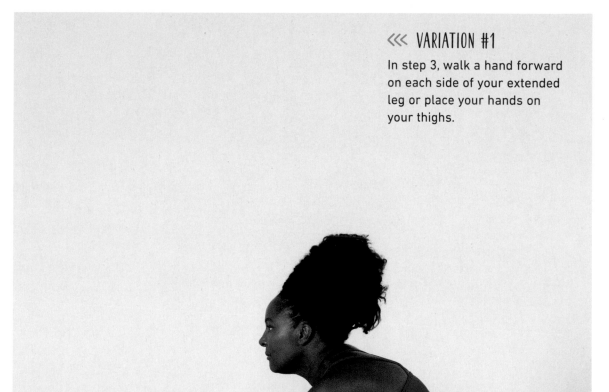

⟪ VARIATION #1

In step 3, walk a hand forward on each side of your extended leg or place your hands on your thighs.

FLEX YOUR FEET
TOWARD YOUR BODY

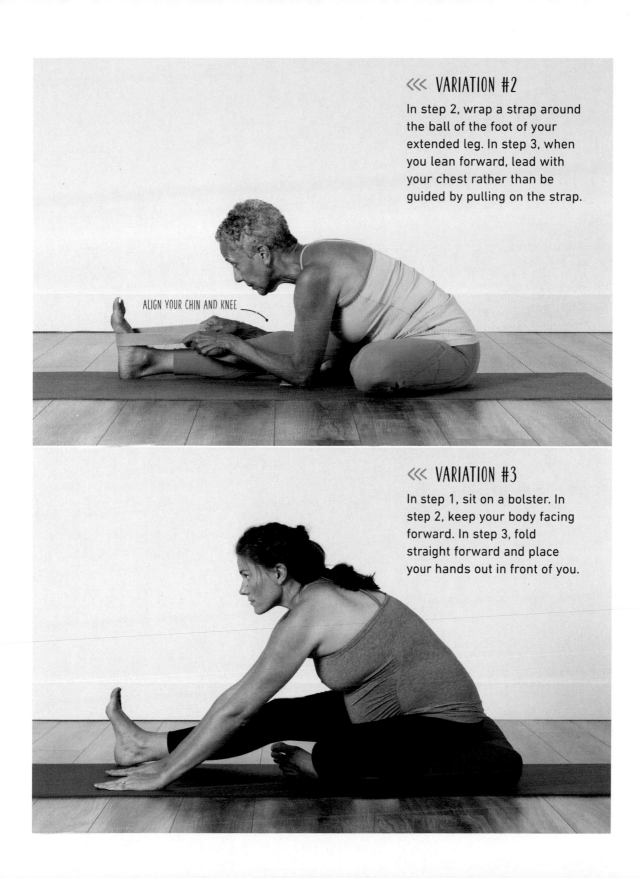

⋘ VARIATION #2

In step 2, wrap a strap around the ball of the foot of your extended leg. In step 3, when you lean forward, lead with your chest rather than be guided by pulling on the strap.

ALIGN YOUR CHIN AND KNEE

⋘ VARIATION #3

In step 1, sit on a bolster. In step 2, keep your body facing forward. In step 3, fold straight forward and place your hands out in front of you.

Revolved Side Angle

>>> PARSVAKONASANA <<<

This twist starts from under your rib cage and the flexibility of your clavicle and scapula aids in the upper-body stretch. This pose builds strength and balance in your legs while also stimulating your lungs and abdominal organs.

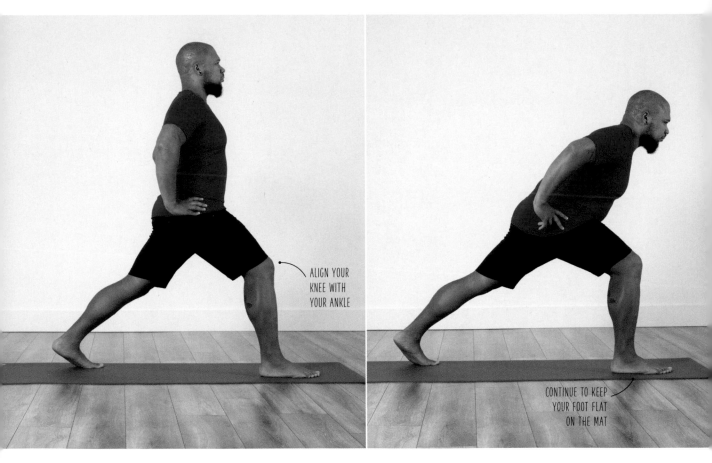

ALIGN YOUR KNEE WITH YOUR ANKLE

CONTINUE TO KEEP YOUR FOOT FLAT ON THE MAT

1 Stand in the middle of the mat, step your right leg forward, and keep your right foot flat. Step your left leg behind you and lift your left heel. Face your torso toward the top of the mat and place your hands on your hips.

2 Bend at your waist and lean forward until your shoulders align with your right knee.

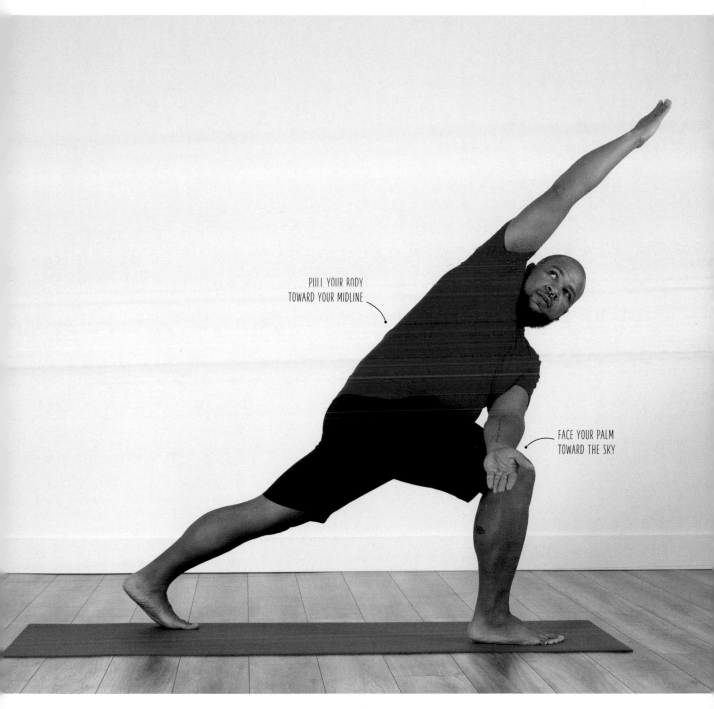

PULL YOUR BODY
TOWARD YOUR MIDLINE

FACE YOUR PALM
TOWARD THE SKY

3 Rotate your torso toward your right thigh. Place your left elbow on the outside of your right knee and press your forearm against your right thigh. Extend your right arm until aligned with your left leg. Hold this position for 3 to 5 full breaths. Repeat these steps on the other side.

～REVOLVED SIDE ANGLE～
VARIATIONS

This pose can prove challenging if you have a larger midsection, tight shoulders, or shorter arms. These variations use a block to make the movements easier.

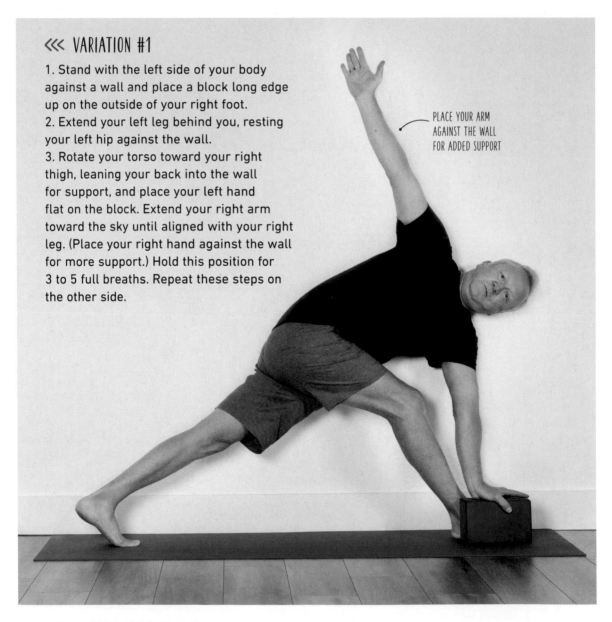

‹‹‹ VARIATION #1

1. Stand with the left side of your body against a wall and place a block long edge up on the outside of your right foot.
2. Extend your left leg behind you, resting your left hip against the wall.
3. Rotate your torso toward your right thigh, leaning your back into the wall for support, and place your left hand flat on the block. Extend your right arm toward the sky until aligned with your right leg. (Place your right hand against the wall for more support.) Hold this position for 3 to 5 full breaths. Repeat these steps on the other side.

PLACE YOUR ARM AGAINST THE WALL FOR ADDED SUPPORT

>>> VARIATION #2

Place a block on the outside of your right leg. In step 3, when you twist, bring your left arm toward the outside of your right foot. Place your left hand on the block and extend your right arm toward the sky until aligned with your right leg.

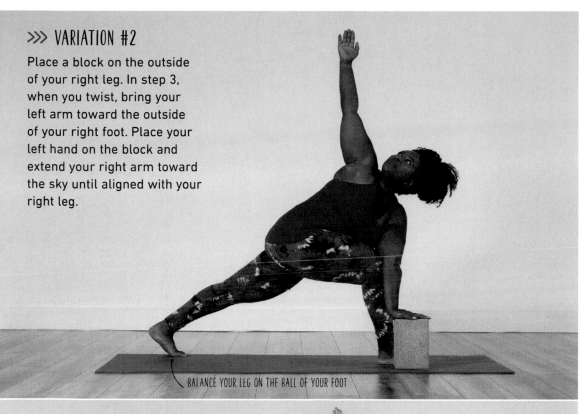

BALANCE YOUR LEG ON THE BALL OF YOUR FOOT

>>> VARIATION #3

In step 1, place your right knee on the mat and a block on the inside of your left leg. In step 2, when you twist, place your left hand on the block and extend your right arm toward the sky or rest your right hand on your hip.

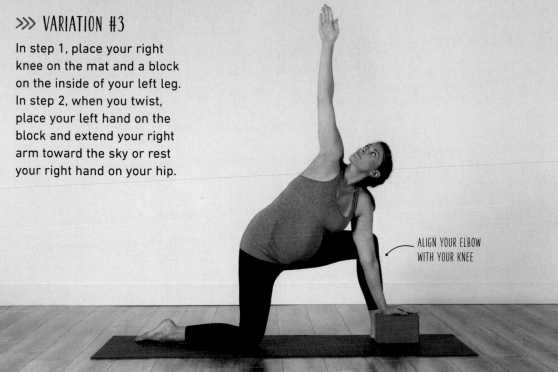

ALIGN YOUR ELBOW WITH YOUR KNEE

Wind Relieving

>>> PAWANMUKTASANA <<<

This supine pose helps massage your abdominal organs and encourages the release of tension in your belly and lower back. And as the name suggests, this pose can also aid with digestion.

1 Lie on your back, with your legs extended and your arms relaxed at your sides.

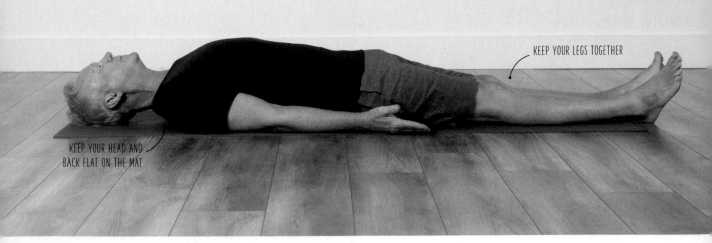

KEEP YOUR LEGS TOGETHER

KEEP YOUR HEAD AND BACK FLAT ON THE MAT

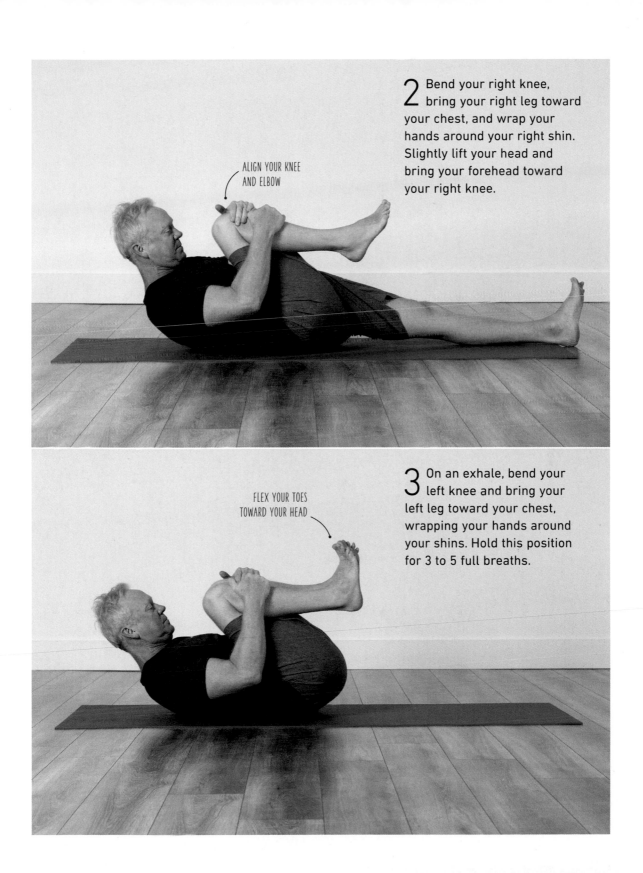

2 Bend your right knee, bring your right leg toward your chest, and wrap your hands around your right shin. Slightly lift your head and bring your forehead toward your right knee.

ALIGN YOUR KNEE AND ELBOW

3 On an exhale, bend your left knee and bring your left leg toward your chest, wrapping your hands around your shins. Hold this position for 3 to 5 full breaths.

FLEX YOUR TOES TOWARD YOUR HEAD

VARIATIONS

If you have an abundance in the center of your body,
this might be a difficult pose. But worry not: There are
a couple variations you can perform instead.

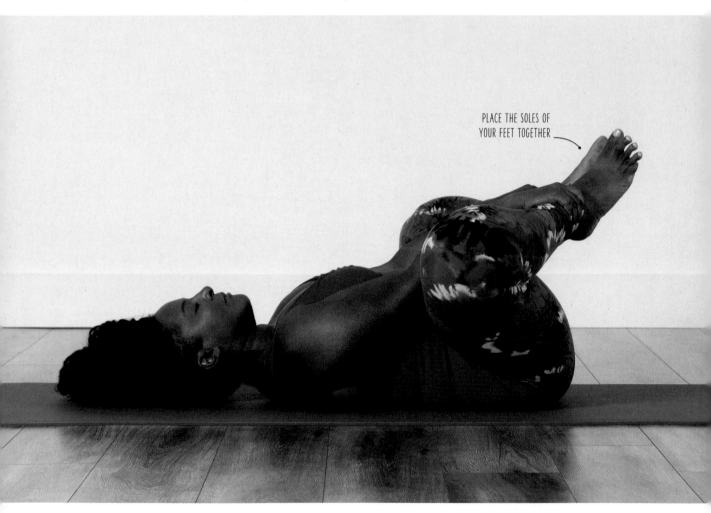

PLACE THE SOLES OF
YOUR FEET TOGETHER

>>> VARIATION #1

In step 3, bring your knees toward
your armpits, allowing your knees
to fall open, and grab your ankles
with your hands.

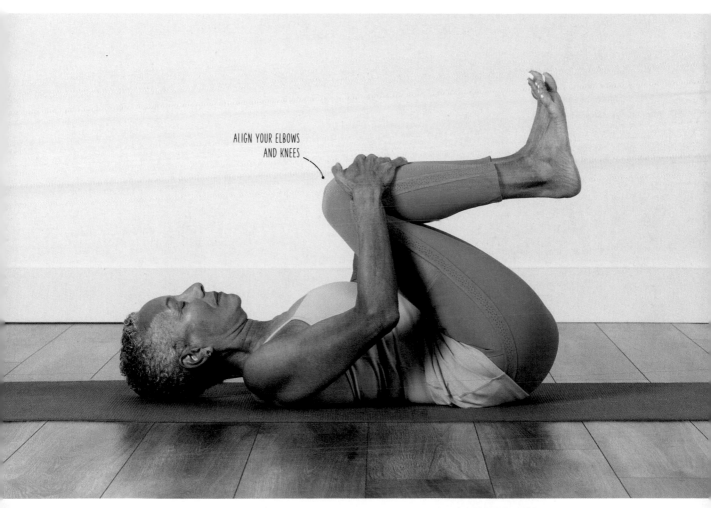

ALIGN YOUR ELBOWS
AND KNEES

>>> VARIATION #2

In steps 2 and 3, keep your head
flat on the mat.

Yoga Squat

>>>MALASANA<<<

This is no ordinary squat. It's a powerful pose that stretches your inner thighs and hip flexors while also strengthening your lower back and leg muscles. Engaging your abdominal muscles helps you maintain your balance.

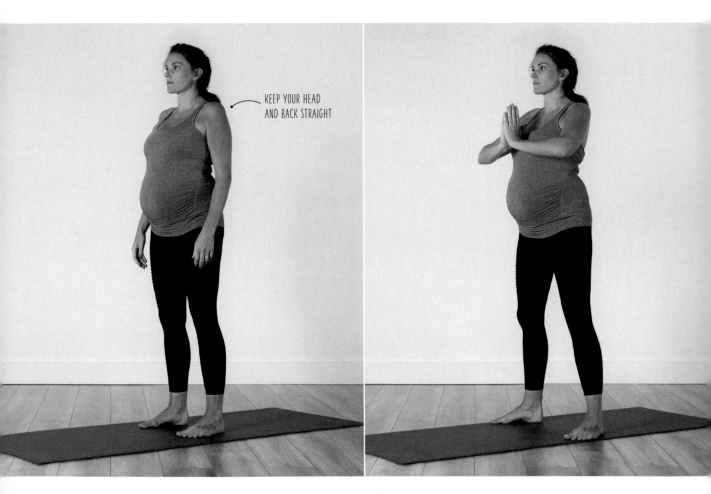

KEEP YOUR HEAD AND BACK STRAIGHT

1 Stand in the middle of the mat, with your weight balanced equally between your feet and your arms relaxed at your sides.

2 Place your feet as wide as the mat, angling your feet toward the corners of the top of the mat. Place your hands on your hips or in a prayer position in front of your chest.

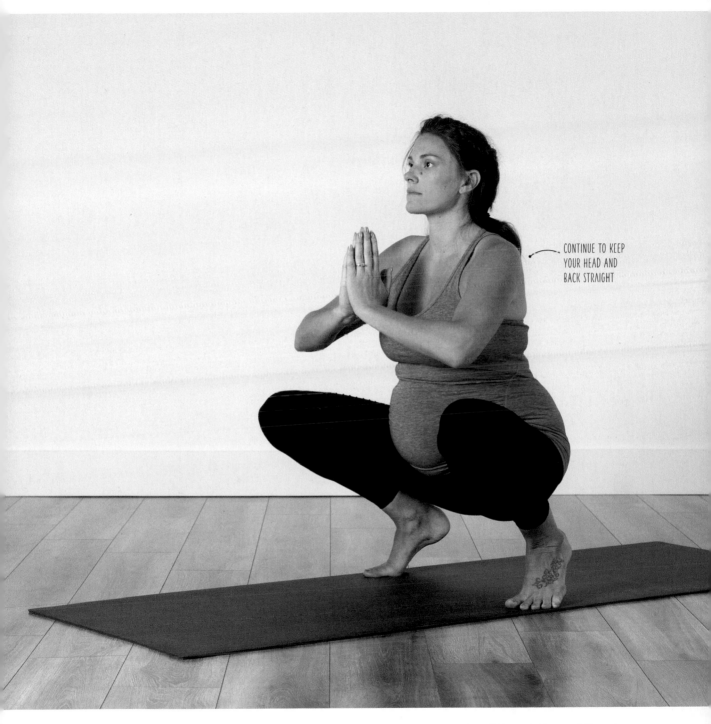

CONTINUE TO KEEP
YOUR HEAD AND
BACK STRAIGHT

3 Bend your knees to lower yourself into a squat. Lift onto
your toes or widen your feet until your heels touch the
mat. (If you lift onto your toes, you can place a folded blanket
under your heels.) Hold this position for 3 to 5 full breaths.

∽ YOGA SQUAT ∾
VARIATIONS

This squat can put a lot of pressure on your knee joints.
Using a prop can help relieve some of this pressure as you
lower into the squat and as you hold that position.

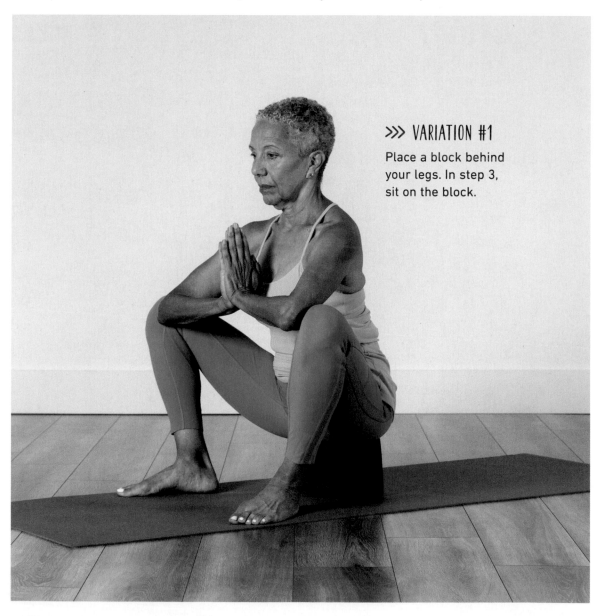

>>> VARIATION #1
Place a block behind
your legs. In step 3,
sit on the block.

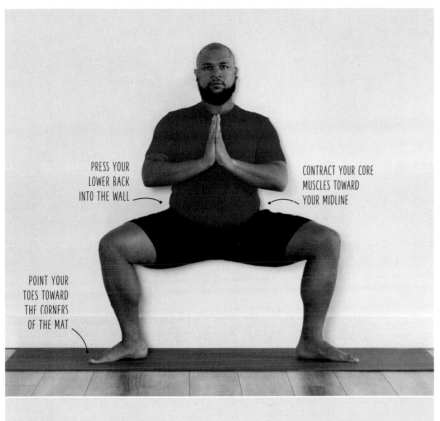

PRESS YOUR LOWER BACK INTO THE WALL

CONTRACT YOUR CORE MUSCLES TOWARD YOUR MIDLINE

POINT YOUR TOES TOWARD THE CORNERS OF THE MAT

>>> VARIATION #2

1. Stand with your back against a wall and your arms relaxed at your sides.
2. Widen your stance, bend your knees, and slide your back down the wall until you're in a squatting position. Relax your arms at your sides, place your hands in a prayer position in front of your chest, or rest your hands on your thighs. Hold this position for 3 to 5 full breaths.

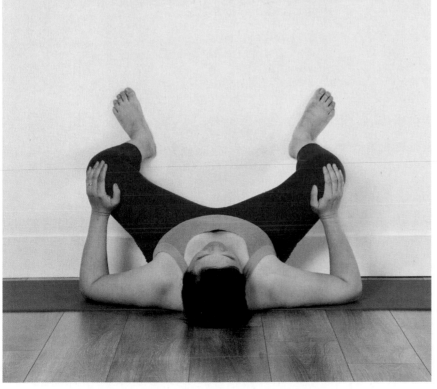

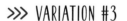

>>> VARIATION #3

1. Facing a wall, lie on your back, with your knees bent and your feet flat against the wall.
2. Angle your feet to resemble a squatting position. (If your legs need more space, move farther away from the wall.) Relax your arms at your sides, place your hands in a prayer position in front of your chest, or rest your hands on your thighs. Hold this position for 3 to 5 full breaths.

DYLAN

WHO IS DYLAN GALOS?

I'm a dreamer and a realist, a lover and a fighter, someone who wades through the world searching for certainty and accepting relativity. I live in the spaces between categories and labels, and I find truth in paradox. Based on impressions from the outside, one might be surprised I'm a big nerdy yoga teacher who loves to play with puppies and cats. I love bad puns, drone metal, and rainbows.

I'm also an epidemiologist (meaning I study the determinants of health and health-related states and events at a population level). I work at an evaluation and research firm working on projects that focus on the social systems and behaviors that influence our health, evaluating programs, creating policies, and working with practitioners. I also teach at universities as an adjunct professor—when time permits.

HOW DOES YOGA HELP YOU COMBAT OBSTACLES IN YOUR LIFE—PHYSICAL, MENTAL, AND EMOTIONAL?

Learning to be more patient and learning how and when to stay in uncomfortable situations. Not only that but also to discern whether there's value in them. I've learned that walking away from something is sometimes not only a necessary choice but also a wise one. The biggest obstacle that yoga has taught me to face is the notion of seeking and clinging to the idea of something permanent; nothing is permanent. What I've learned from yoga is that while everything changes, there is something familiar and grounding that can be found in the situations life throws our way.

FAVORITE POSE
>>> REVOLVING HALF MOON

MOST CHALLENGING POSE
>>> SIDE CROW

OCCUPATION
>>> EPIDEMIOLOGIST

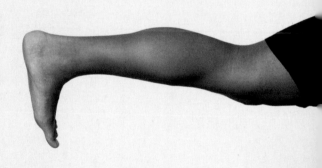

HOW DID YOGA BECOME A PART OF YOUR LIFE? HOW HAVE YOU SUSTAINED YOUR PRACTICE?

It wasn't until I was in a motorcycle crash in 2012 that I began to explore a practice with consistency and inquire more about the aspects of yoga that are off the mat. Yoga changed my life by giving me a space to find consistency and contentment without requiring anything besides my body. My practice has helped me have fewer walls to different kinds of people and to be more open. That's not to say practicing yoga automatically makes someone a kind person, but rather, it's been a set of tools that's given me space to make changes and be.

Yoga is so much more than a Google search tells you it is. You don't ever have to stand on your hands to do yoga, and while not everyone will find that yoga is the thing for them, I believe there's a practice of yoga that can be reached by everyone. At some point—and I hear this is common—I've become less strict about the specifics of what my yoga practice looks like. It's more important to be consistent with it in a way that fits. Rarely does my practice look like a 75-minute group class in a studio. A lot of it is bringing yoga to the other things I do. Sometimes, it involves bringing that same focus and attention to the weight room with barbells; other times, it involves lying down on bolsters. What I've learned from allowing flexibility in my yoga practice is that it makes it possible to be consistent.

Fire Log

>>> AGNISTAMBHASANA <<<

This powerful hip-opening pose is known for building heat within the body, especially an intense stretch in your hip flexors. These movements can also invigorate your outer hips, thighs, buttocks, lower back, and internal organs.

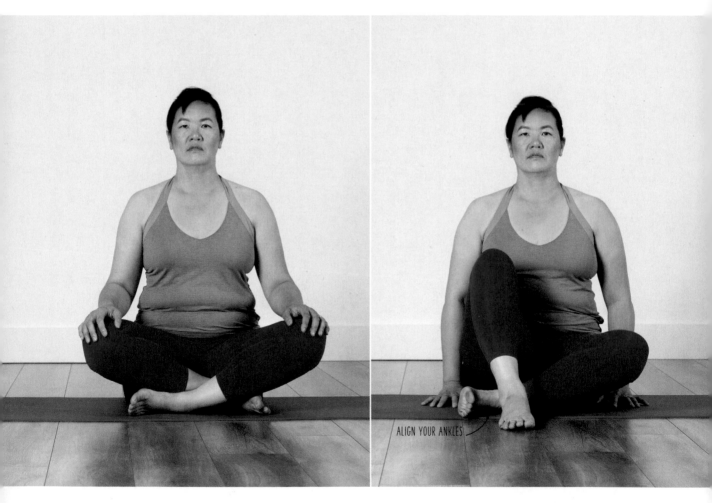

ALIGN YOUR ANKLES

1 Sit in a cross-legged position, with your hands resting on your knees. (You can also sit on a folded blanket for more support.)

2 Step your right foot forward and slide your left heel toward your sitting bones, placing your hands at your sides.

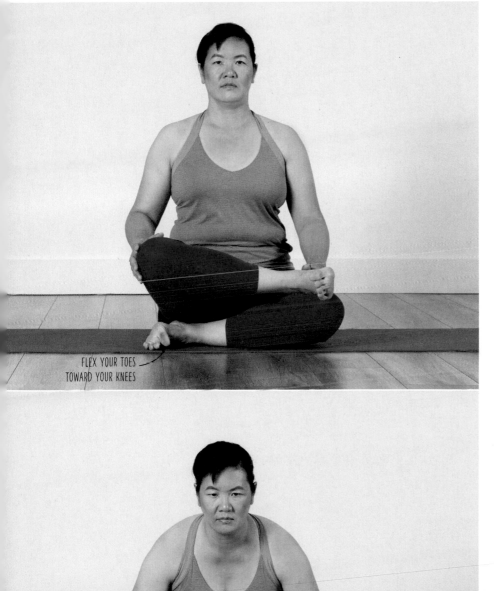

FLEX YOUR TOES
TOWARD YOUR KNEES

3 Place your right foot on top of your left knee, grab your right foot with your left hand, and rest your right hand on your right knee.

KEEP YOUR SHINS PARALLEL
WITH THE SIDES OF THE MAT

4 Press your tailbone down into the mat, lengthening your spine, and bend at your waist and lean your chest over your legs. Hold this position for 3 to 5 full breaths.

⌒ FIRE LOG ⌒
VARIATIONS

There's more than one way to build a fire. And if you have
or had an injury to your hips and knees, you might want
to try one of the variations of this pose.

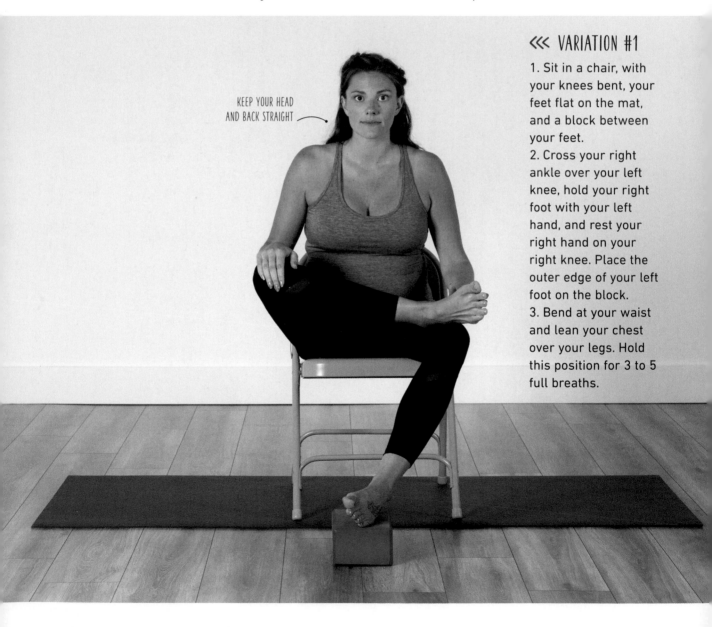

KEEP YOUR HEAD
AND BACK STRAIGHT

⟪⟪ VARIATION #1

1. Sit in a chair, with your knees bent, your feet flat on the mat, and a block between your feet.
2. Cross your right ankle over your left knee, hold your right foot with your left hand, and rest your right hand on your right knee. Place the outer edge of your left foot on the block.
3. Bend at your waist and lean your chest over your legs. Hold this position for 3 to 5 full breaths.

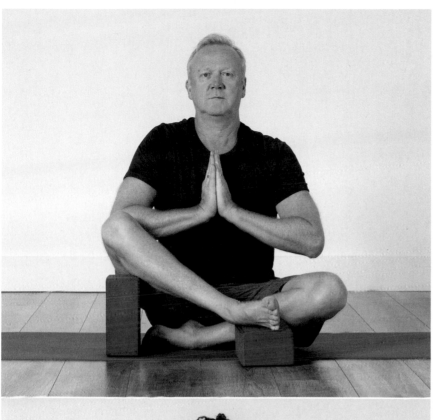

⋘ VARIATION #2

Place a block long side up on the mat near your left leg and place a block short edge up near your right leg. In step 2, place your right foot on the flat block and place your knee on the tall block. (You can also place the block under your left foot instead.) Bring your hands together in a prayer position in front of your chest.

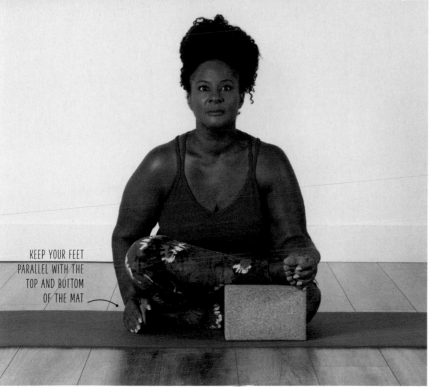

KEEP YOUR FEET PARALLEL WITH THE TOP AND BOTTOM OF THE MAT

⋘ VARIATION #3

Place a block longest edge up near your left leg. In step 2, place your right foot on the block and place your right hand on the sole of your left foot.

Dancer

>>>NATARAJASANA<<<

It's time to show off your dance moves! And while you're doing that, you can increase strength and flexibility; relieve tightness in your shoulders, chest, and hips; develop your thigh muscles; and improve your overall balance and focus.

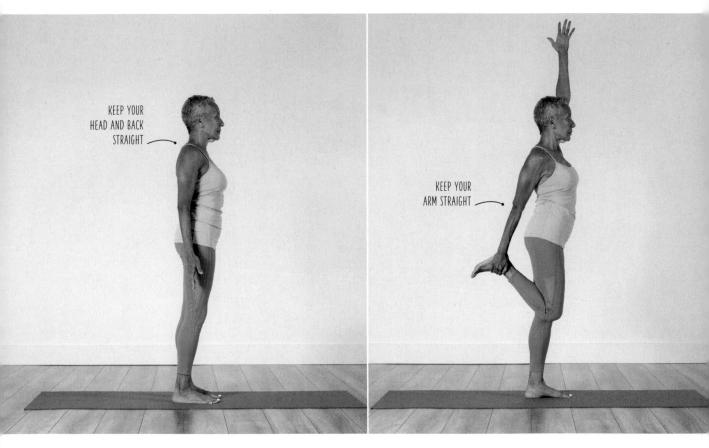

KEEP YOUR HEAD AND BACK STRAIGHT

KEEP YOUR ARM STRAIGHT

1 Stand in the middle of the mat, with your weight balanced equally between your feet and your arms relaxed at your sides.

2 Bend your right knee and lift your right heel toward your buttocks. Grab your right ankle with your right hand, shifting your weight to your left foot, and extend your left arm toward the sky.

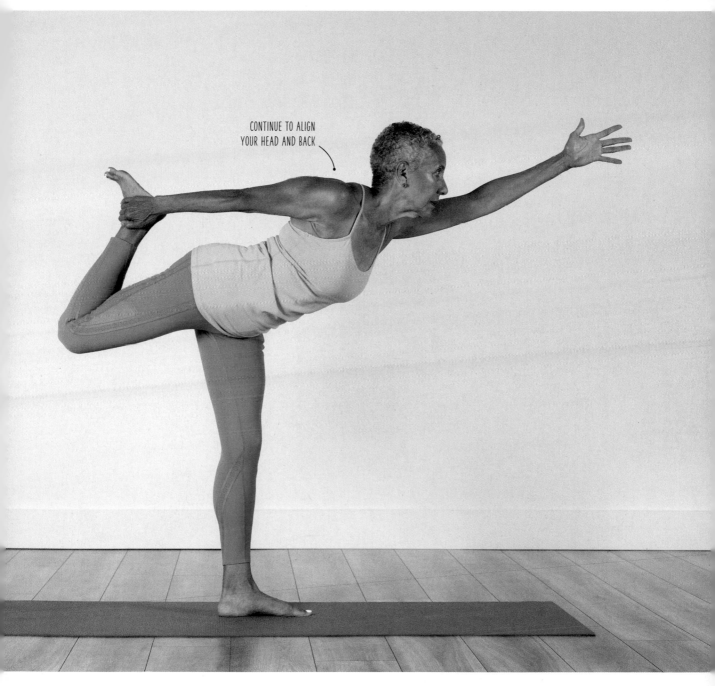

CONTINUE TO ALIGN
YOUR HEAD AND BACK

3 Bend at your waist and slowly lean forward
until your left arm aligns with your right
leg. Lift your right leg up as far as you can and
press your right foot into your right hand. Hold
this position for 3 to 5 full breaths. Repeat these
steps on the other side.

DANCER

VARIATIONS

There's more than one way to dance. These variations use a strap, a wall, or the mat to help make this pose more accessible—and more fun for your body.

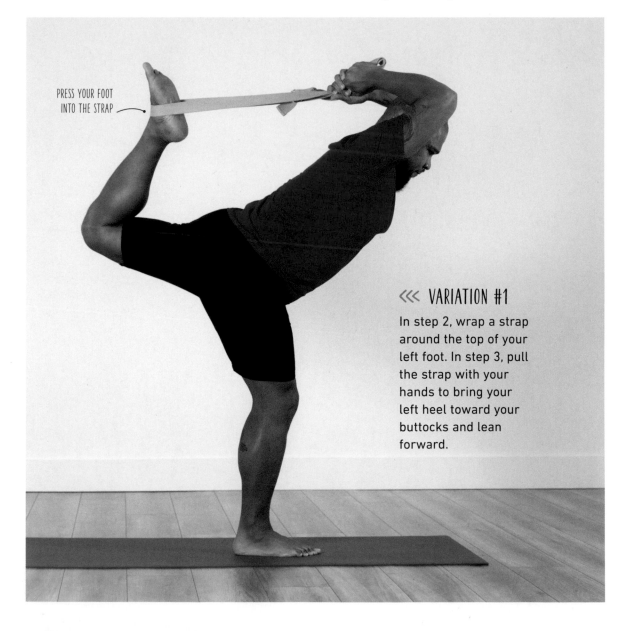

PRESS YOUR FOOT INTO THE STRAP

⫸ VARIATION #1

In step 2, wrap a strap around the top of your left foot. In step 3, pull the strap with your hands to bring your left heel toward your buttocks and lean forward.

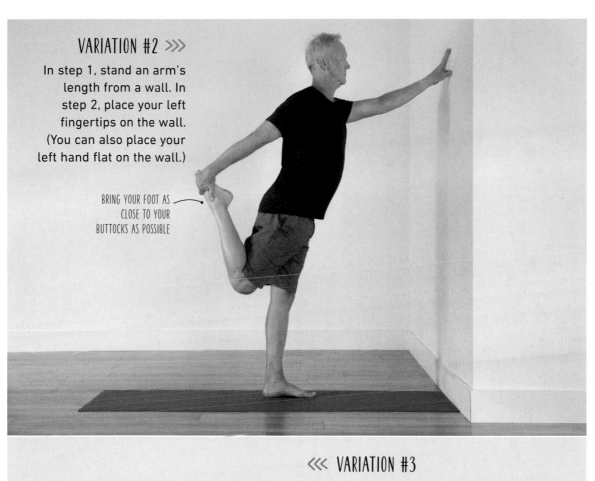

VARIATION #2 >>>

In step 1, stand an arm's length from a wall. In step 2, place your left fingertips on the wall. (You can also place your left hand flat on the wall.)

BRING YOUR FOOT AS CLOSE TO YOUR BUTTOCKS AS POSSIBLE

<<< VARIATION #3

1. Lie on your belly, with your legs extended and your hands and forearms flat on the floor near your head.
2. Bend your right knee, reach your right arm behind you, and grab your right ankle with your right hand. Hold this position for 3 to 5 full breaths. Repeat these steps with your left leg.

KEEP YOUR KNEES FLAT ON THE MAT

Half Moon

>>> ARDHA CHANDRASANA <<<

From challenging your balance, building strength in your legs, and stretching your glutes, shoulders, and hips, this pose can impact your entire body. These movements are also great for warming up your muscles.

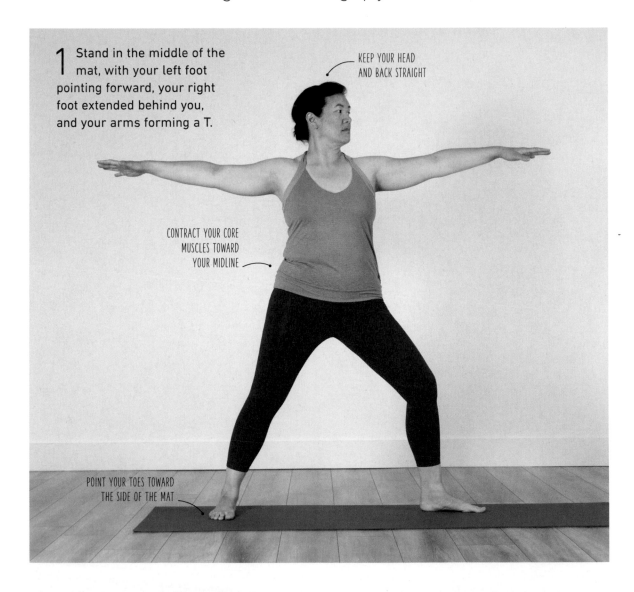

1 Stand in the middle of the mat, with your left foot pointing forward, your right foot extended behind you, and your arms forming a T.

KEEP YOUR HEAD AND BACK STRAIGHT

CONTRACT YOUR CORE MUSCLES TOWARD YOUR MIDLINE

POINT YOUR TOES TOWARD THE SIDE OF THE MAT

2 Bend at your waist toward your left and place your left fingertips on the mat in front of your left foot. Place your right hand on your waist and keep your gaze toward the mat.

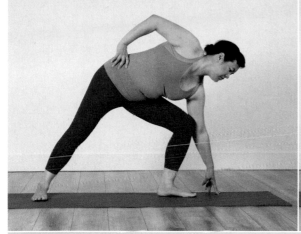

3 Walk your left fingers forward and lift your right leg until parallel with the mat. Place your right fingertips on the mat for extra balance.

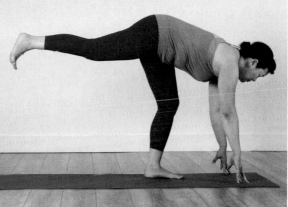

4 Rotate your hips to turn your torso toward your right. Keep your left fingertips on the mat and extend your right arm toward the sky until aligned with your left arm. Hold this position for 3 to 5 full breaths. Repeat these steps on the other side.

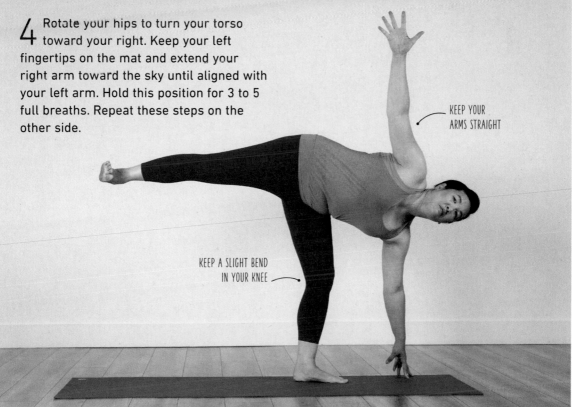

KEEP YOUR ARMS STRAIGHT

KEEP A SLIGHT BEND IN YOUR KNEE

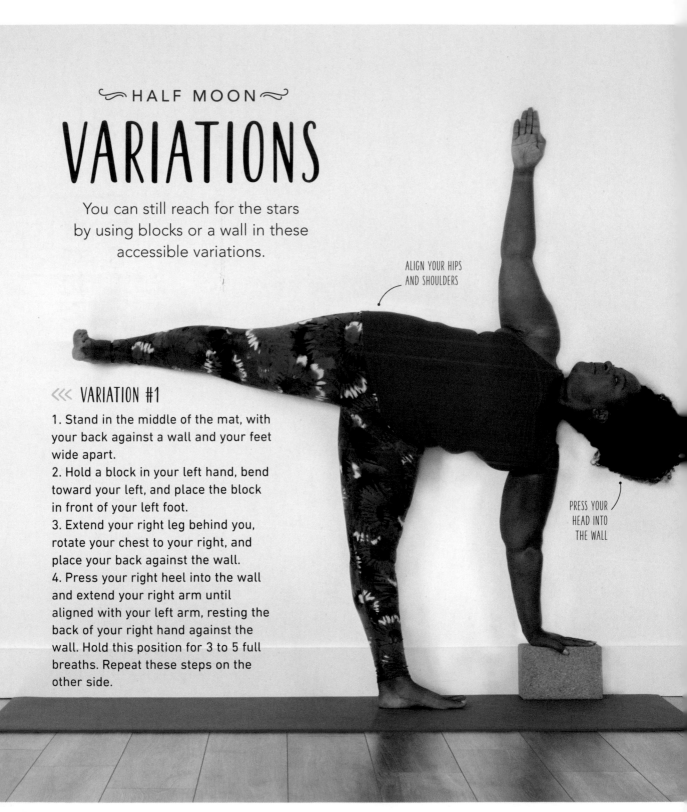

~ HALF MOON ~
VARIATIONS

You can still reach for the stars by using blocks or a wall in these accessible variations.

ALIGN YOUR HIPS AND SHOULDERS

PRESS YOUR HEAD INTO THE WALL

⫷ VARIATION #1

1. Stand in the middle of the mat, with your back against a wall and your feet wide apart.
2. Hold a block in your left hand, bend toward your left, and place the block in front of your left foot.
3. Extend your right leg behind you, rotate your chest to your right, and place your back against the wall.
4. Press your right heel into the wall and extend your right arm until aligned with your left arm, resting the back of your right hand against the wall. Hold this position for 3 to 5 full breaths. Repeat these steps on the other side.

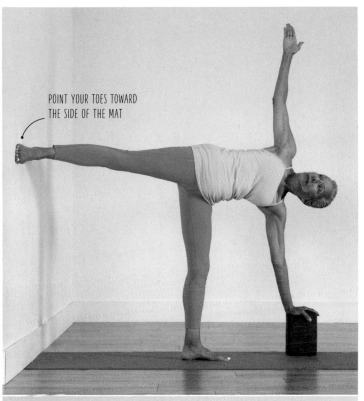

POINT YOUR TOES TOWARD
THE SIDE OF THE MAT

‹‹‹ VARIATION #2

1. Stand facing a couple feet away from a wall, placing a block in front of your left foot.
2. Bend at your waist, extend your right leg behind you, place your right foot flat on the wall, and place your left hand on the block.
3. Rotate your hips to your right, extending your right arm toward the sky until aligned with your left arm, and press your left hand into the block. Hold this position for 3 to 5 full breaths. Repeat these steps on the other side.

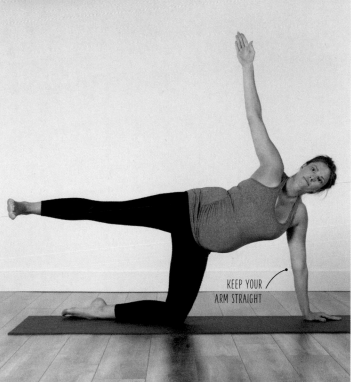

KEEP YOUR
ARM STRAIGHT

‹‹‹ VARIATION #3

1. Place your hands, knees, and the tops of your feet flat on the mat.
2. Extend your right leg behind you, keeping your knee straight.
3. Rotate your hips to your right and lift your right arm and right leg off the mat. Extend your right arm toward the sky until aligned with your left arm. Hold this position for 3 to 5 full breaths. Repeat these steps on the other side.

Boat

>>> NAVASANA <<<

It's time to float toward strengthening your core muscles, especially your hip flexors, abdominals, and lower back. This adventure can also help you find physical balance by continually engaging your abs and focusing on your breath.

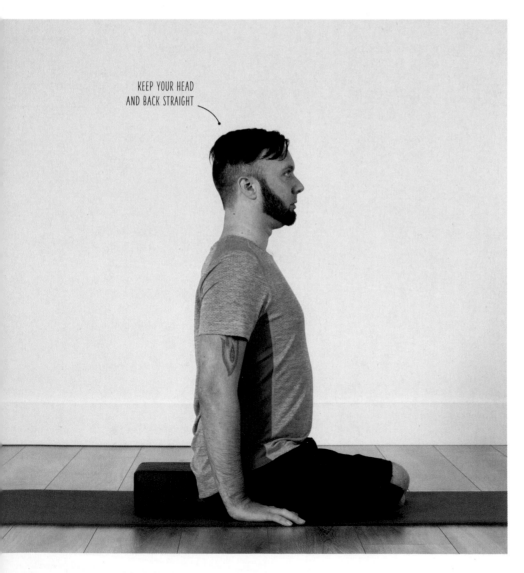

KEEP YOUR HEAD AND BACK STRAIGHT

1 Sit in the middle of the mat, with your legs extended and your arms relaxed at your sides. (You can place a block behind your lower back for added support.)

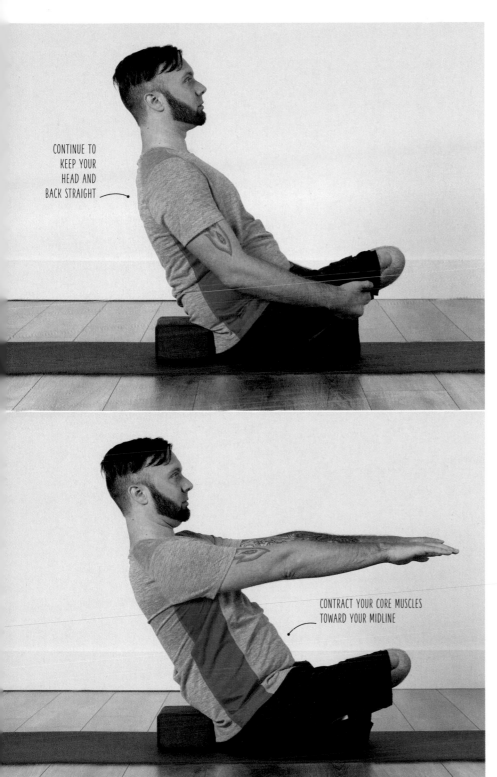

CONTINUE TO
KEEP YOUR
HEAD AND
BACK STRAIGHT

2 Shift your weight to the back of your sitting bones, making sure to not roll onto your tailbone. Slightly bend your elbows and place your hands behind your thighs.

CONTRACT YOUR CORE MUSCLES
TOWARD YOUR MIDLINE

3 Lean backward, lift your legs off the mat, and extend your arms until parallel with the mat. Hold this position for 3 to 5 full breaths.

⌒ BOAT ⌒
VARIATIONS

You might sometimes need a lifeboat. Try these variations
to help make this pose more accessible and to enjoy
smooth sailing in your yoga practice.

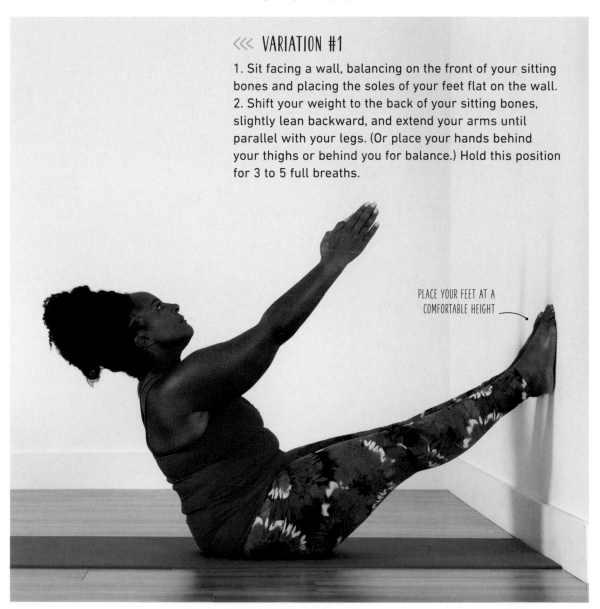

⟨⟨⟨ VARIATION #1

1. Sit facing a wall, balancing on the front of your sitting
bones and placing the soles of your feet flat on the wall.
2. Shift your weight to the back of your sitting bones,
slightly lean backward, and extend your arms until
parallel with your legs. (Or place your hands behind
your thighs or behind you for balance.) Hold this position
for 3 to 5 full breaths.

PLACE YOUR FEET AT A
COMFORTABLE HEIGHT

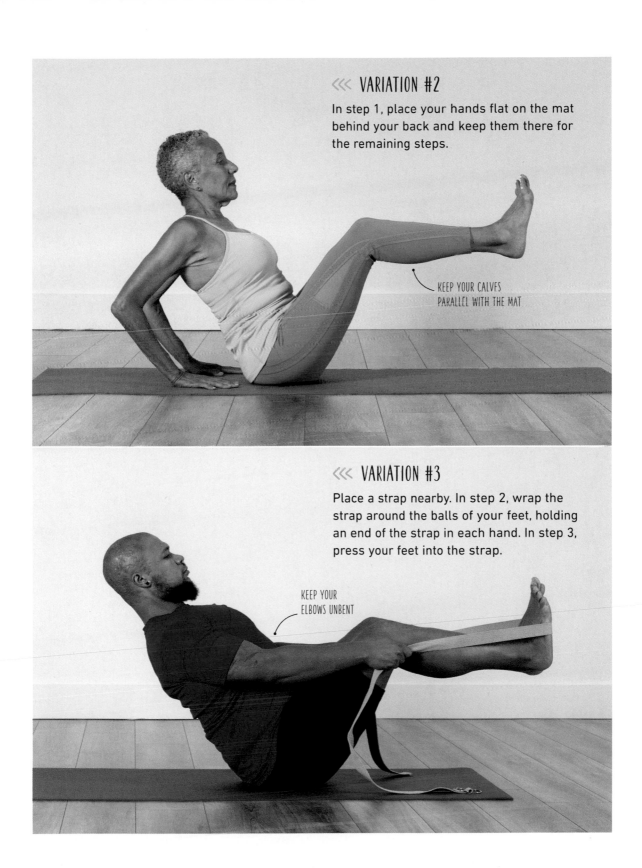

««« VARIATION #2

In step 1, place your hands flat on the mat behind your back and keep them there for the remaining steps.

KEEP YOUR CALVES PARALLEL WITH THE MAT

««« VARIATION #3

Place a strap nearby. In step 2, wrap the strap around the balls of your feet, holding an end of the strap in each hand. In step 3, press your feet into the strap.

KEEP YOUR ELBOWS UNBENT

Tree

>>> VRKSASANA <<<

Performing this pose can help you connect with your core muscles. Not only can these movements increase your balance and stability, but they can also challenge your body to depend on your brain's mental focus.

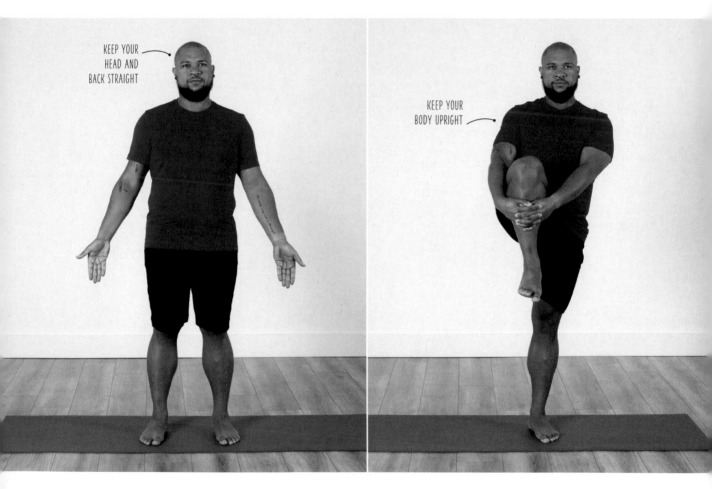

KEEP YOUR HEAD AND BACK STRAIGHT

KEEP YOUR BODY UPRIGHT

1 Stand in the middle of the mat, with your weight balanced equally between your feet and your arms relaxed at your sides.

2 Shift your weight to your left foot, slowly bend your right knee, and bring your right knee into your chest.

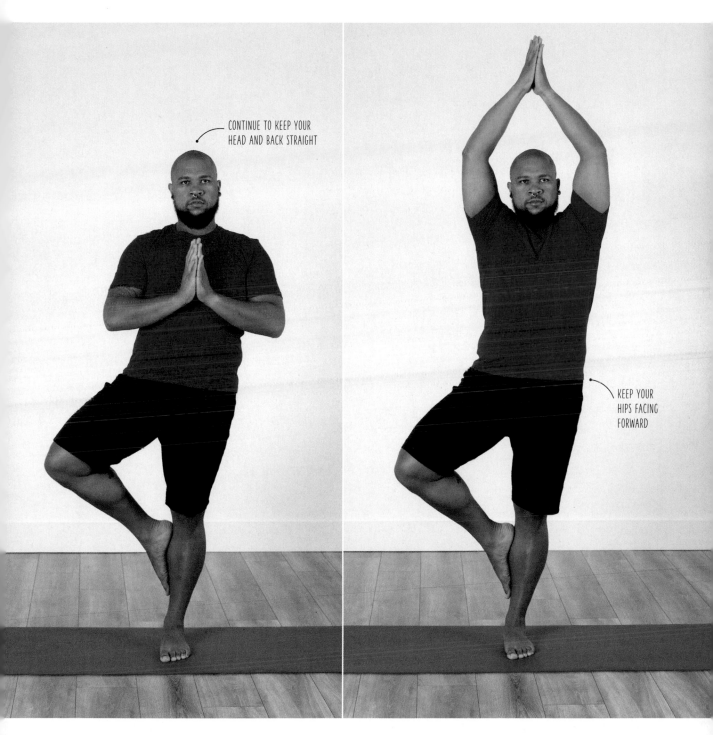

CONTINUE TO KEEP YOUR
HEAD AND BACK STRAIGHT

KEEP YOUR
HIPS FACING
FORWARD

3 Place the sole of your right foot on the inside of your left calf or thigh, pull your legs to the midline of your body, and place your hands in a prayer position in front of your chest.

4 When you feel balanced, lift your arms toward the sky, keeping a slight bend in your elbows. Hold this position for 3 to 5 full breaths. Repeat these steps on the other side.

∽ TREE ∽
VARIATIONS

We're always trying to find balance in our lives.
It can be especially challenging in yoga. But these variations
can offer you a way to get closer to centering yourself—
physically and mentally.

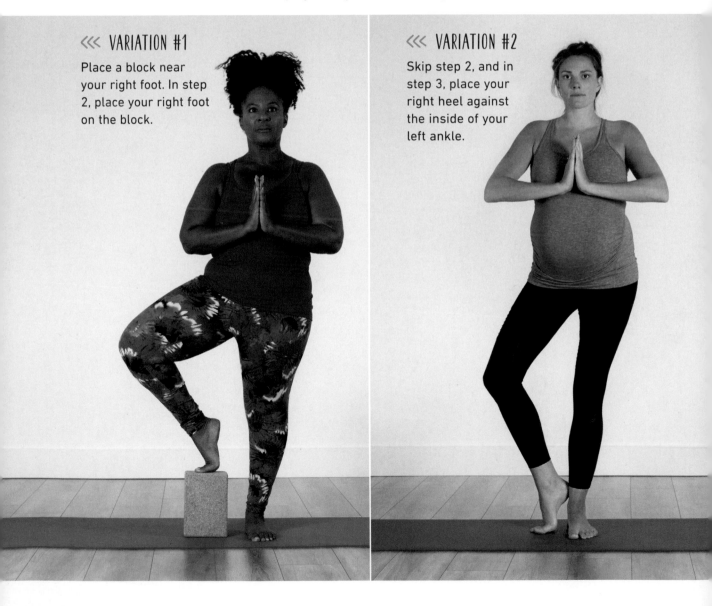

⟪ VARIATION #1

Place a block near
your right foot. In step
2, place your right foot
on the block.

⟪ VARIATION #2

Skip step 2, and in
step 3, place your
right heel against
the inside of your
left ankle.

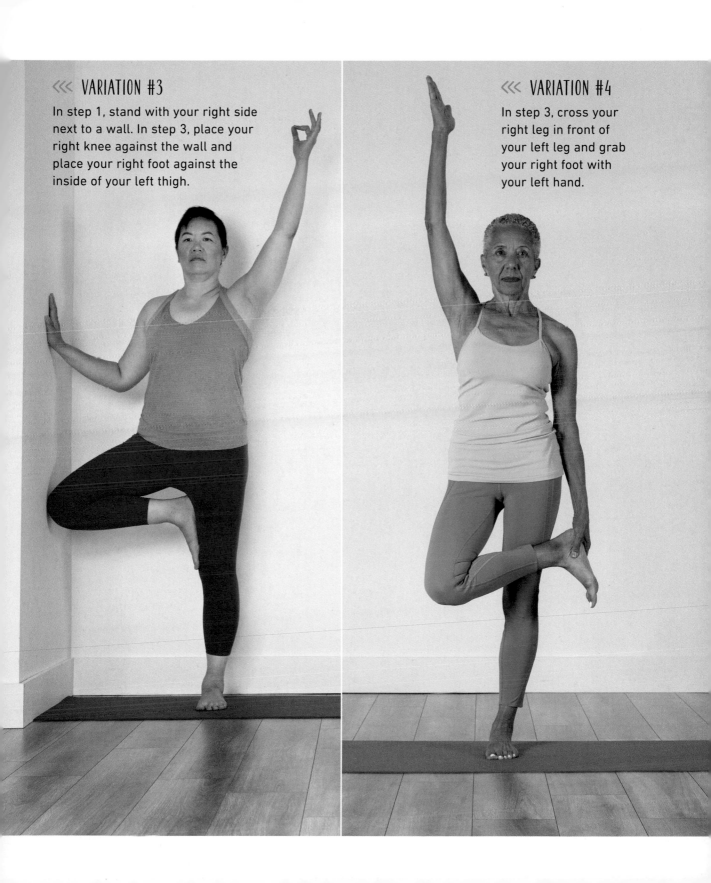

≪ VARIATION #3

In step 1, stand with your right side next to a wall. In step 3, place your right knee against the wall and place your right foot against the inside of your left thigh.

≪ VARIATION #4

In step 3, cross your right leg in front of your left leg and grab your right foot with your left hand.

Triangle

>>> TRIKONASANA <<<

This lateral-facing standing pose opens your hips
and shoulders and stretches your hamstrings. Performing
these movements can also lengthen your torso and help
build balance and strength in your legs.

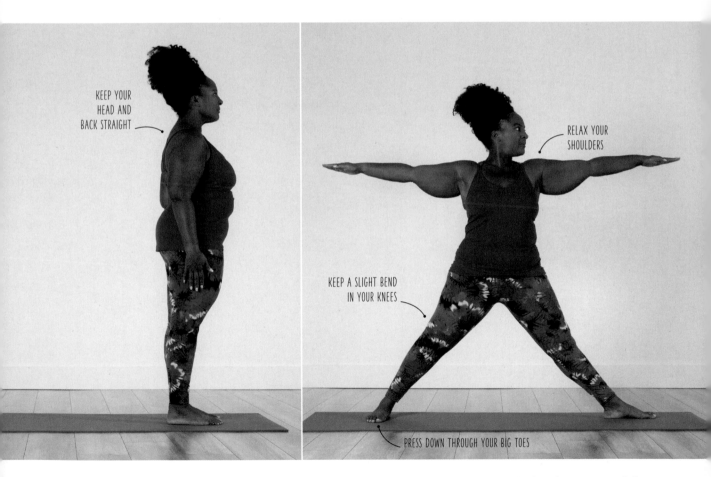

KEEP YOUR
HEAD AND
BACK STRAIGHT

RELAX YOUR
SHOULDERS

KEEP A SLIGHT BEND
IN YOUR KNEES

PRESS DOWN THROUGH YOUR BIG TOES

1 Stand at the top of the mat, with your weight balanced equally between your feet and your arms relaxed at your sides.

2 Extend your right leg behind you, balancing your weight between your feet, and turn your upper body to your right to face the right side of the mat. Place your right foot parallel with the back of the mat and keep your left foot pointing forward. Extend your arms to form a T.

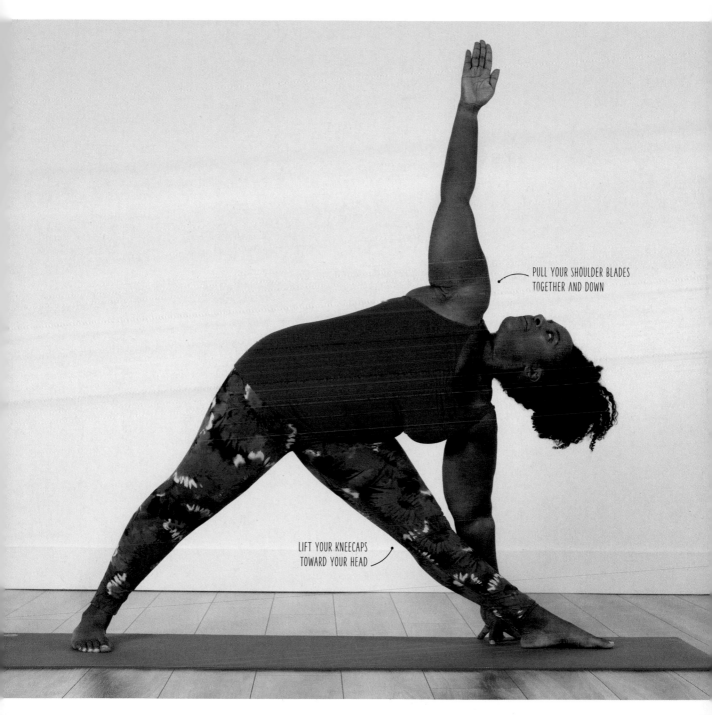

PULL YOUR SHOULDER BLADES
TOGETHER AND DOWN

LIFT YOUR KNEECAPS
TOWARD YOUR HEAD

3 Bend at your left hip and place the fingertips of your left
hand at the outside of your left foot. Rotate your torso to
your right and extend your right arm until aligned with your
left arm. Hold this position for 3 to 5 full breaths. Repeat
these steps on the other side.

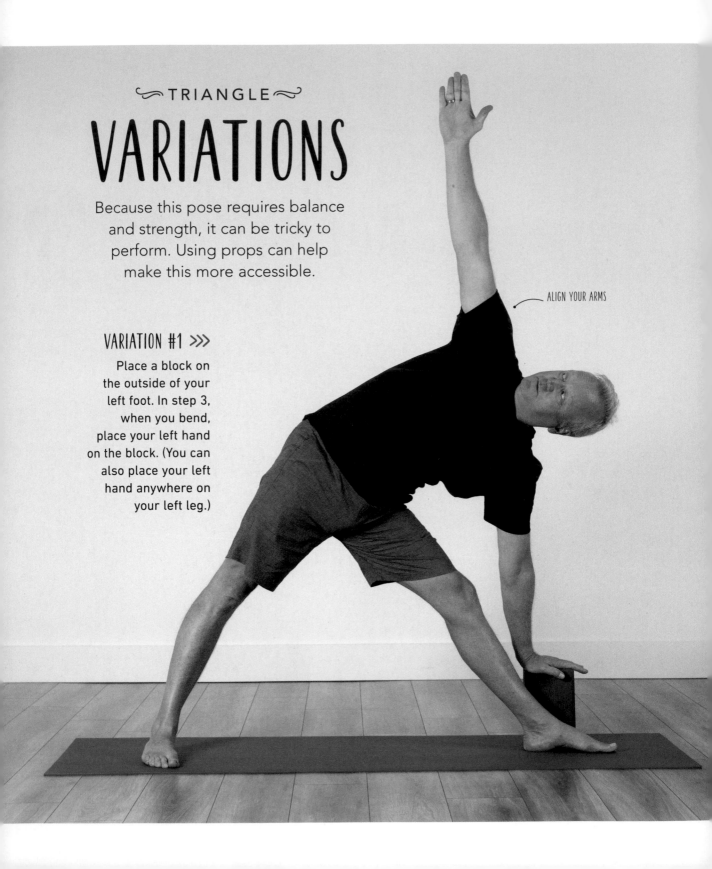

~ TRIANGLE ~

VARIATIONS

Because this pose requires balance and strength, it can be tricky to perform. Using props can help make this more accessible.

ALIGN YOUR ARMS

VARIATION #1 >>>

Place a block on the outside of your left foot. In step 3, when you bend, place your left hand on the block. (You can also place your left hand anywhere on your left leg.)

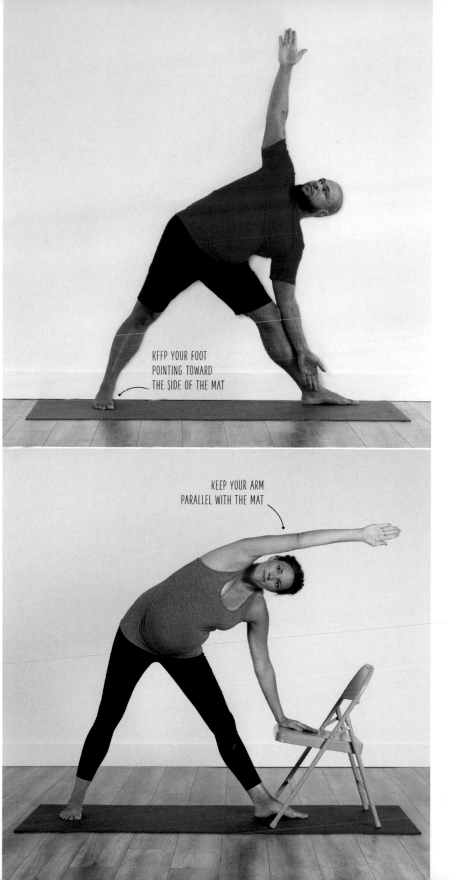

KEEP YOUR FOOT POINTING TOWARD THE SIDE OF THE MAT

KEEP YOUR ARM PARALLEL WITH THE MAT

≪≪ VARIATION #2

1. Stand facing away from a wall, with your right heel pressed into the wall and the outside of your left foot against the wall.
2. Lean backward and place your left hip against the wall.
3. Bend toward your left, touching your left leg with the back of your left hand. Extend your right arm toward the sky until aligned with your left arm. Hold this position for 3 to 5 full breaths. Repeat these steps on the other side.

≪≪ VARIATION #3

In step 1, face the seat of a chair toward you and in front of your left foot. In step 3, place your left hand flat on the seat of the chair and extend your right arm over the back of the chair.

Chair

>>>UTKATASANA<<<

Also known as the Fierce pose because of its intensity, this is great for building strength in your legs. And because this pose's movements have squat-like aspects, you can enjoy similar benefits to that position.

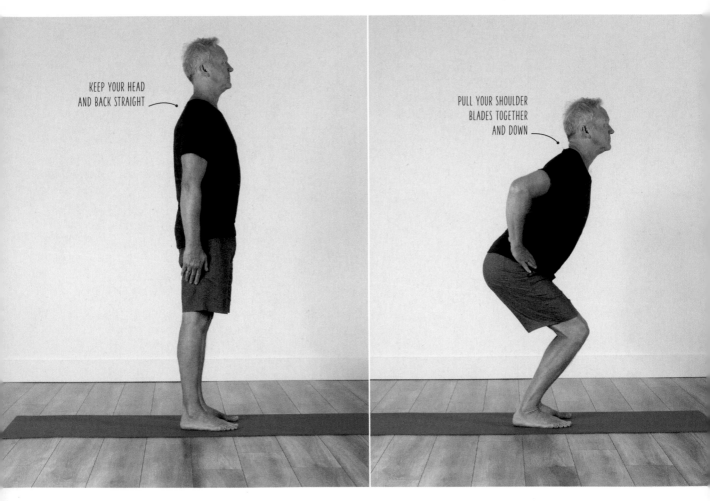

KEEP YOUR HEAD AND BACK STRAIGHT

PULL YOUR SHOULDER BLADES TOGETHER AND DOWN

1 Stand in the middle of the mat, with your weight balanced equally between your feet and your arms relaxed at your sides.

2 On an exhale, bend your knees, shift your weight backward as if lowering yourself into a chair, and place your hands on your waist.

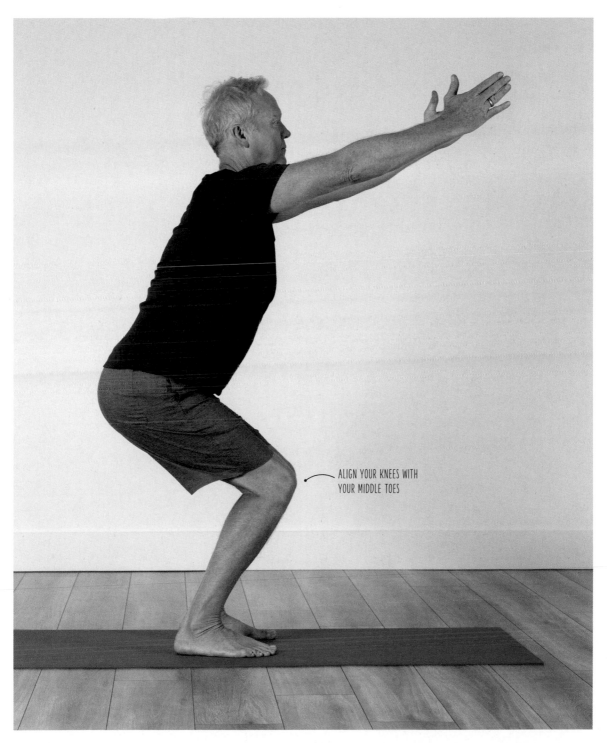

ALIGN YOUR KNEES WITH
YOUR MIDDLE TOES

3 Extend your arms at an angle
toward the sky. Hold this
position for 3 to 5 full breaths.

KEEP YOUR HEAD AND BACK
FLAT AGAINST THE WALL

~ CHAIR ~

VARIATIONS

Because this pose requires tremendous strength in your quads and glutes, you might find it to be too challenging. Try one of these variations that might make the movements more accessible—if not a little easier.

⋘ VARIATION #1

1. Stand facing away from a wall, with your weight balanced equally between your feet and your arms relaxed at your sides.
2. Bend your knees and lean your body against the wall, walking your feet forward until you find a comfortable position.
3. Extend your arms alongside your ears and rest them against the wall. Hold this position for 3 to 5 full breaths.

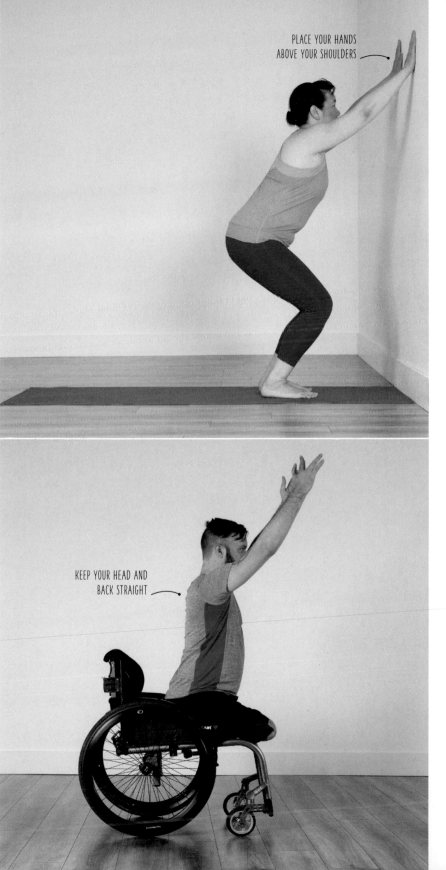

PLACE YOUR HANDS
ABOVE YOUR SHOULDERS

⋘ VARIATION #2

1. Stand facing a wall, with your weight balanced equally between your feet and your arms relaxed at your sides.

2. Bend your knees, shift your weight backward as if lowering yourself into a chair, and place your hands against the wall for support. Hold this position for 3 to 5 full breaths.

KEEP YOUR HEAD AND
BACK STRAIGHT

⋘ VARIATION #3

1. Sit on the edge of a chair, with your feet flat on the floor and your knees aligned with your toes.

2. Extend your arms toward the sky. (You can also place your hands on your knees or place your hands in a prayer position in front of your chest.) Hold this position for 3 to 5 full breaths.

Mountain

>>> TADASANA <<<

Don't let what seems like a simple pose fool you.
It's one of the most common poses in yoga and
a foundational stance for all standing poses. But it's also
the embodiment of standing with intention and integrity.

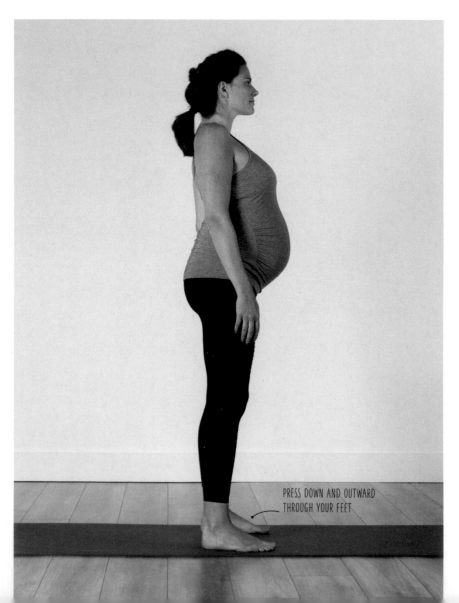

PRESS DOWN AND OUTWARD
THROUGH YOUR FEET

1 Stand in the
middle of the mat,
with your weight
balanced equally
between your feet, the
outer edges of your
feet parallel with the
sides of the mat, and
your arms relaxed at
your sides.

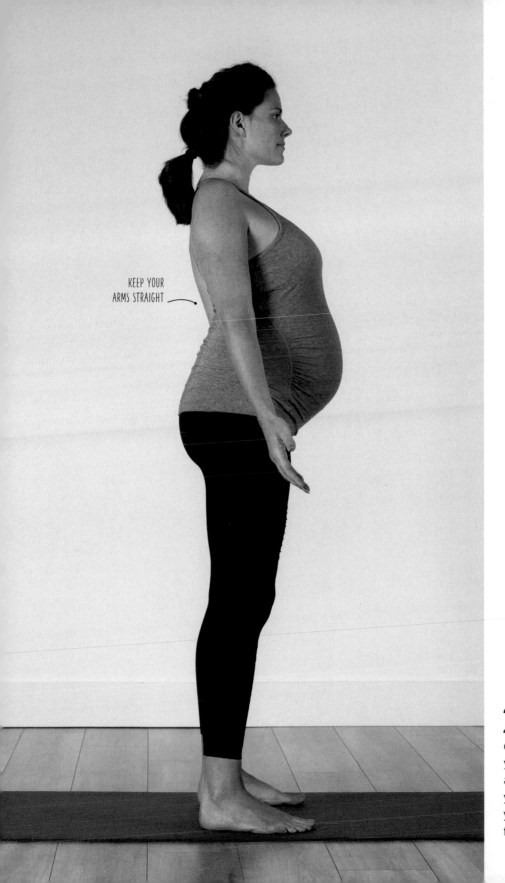

KEEP YOUR
ARMS STRAIGHT

2 Pull your shoulder
blades toward
each other, aligning
your ears, shoulders,
and hips, and turn
your hands away from
you. Hold this position
for 3 to 5 full breaths.

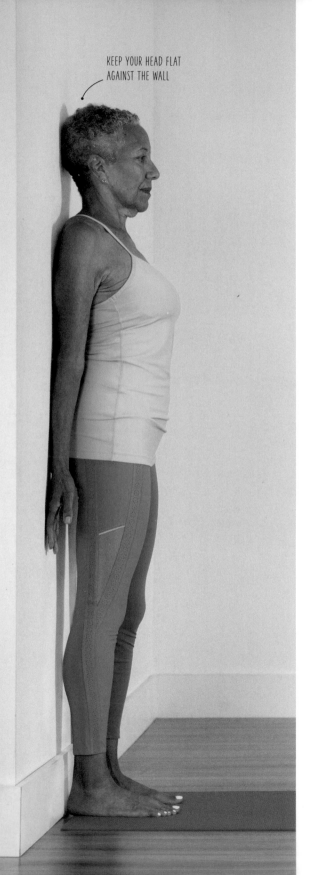

KEEP YOUR HEAD FLAT AGAINST THE WALL

~ MOUNTAIN ~
# VARIATIONS

This pose incorporates a feeling of connection from your feet to your head—a feeling of standing strong. These variations employ similar core principles to the traditional pose.

⫷ VARIATION #1

1. Stand facing away from a wall, with your feet together; your back, heels, sacrum, and shoulder blades flat against the wall; and your arms relaxed at your sides.

2. Pull your shoulder blades toward each other and face your palms forward.

3. Press the backs of your hands into the wall. Hold this position for 3 to 5 full breaths.

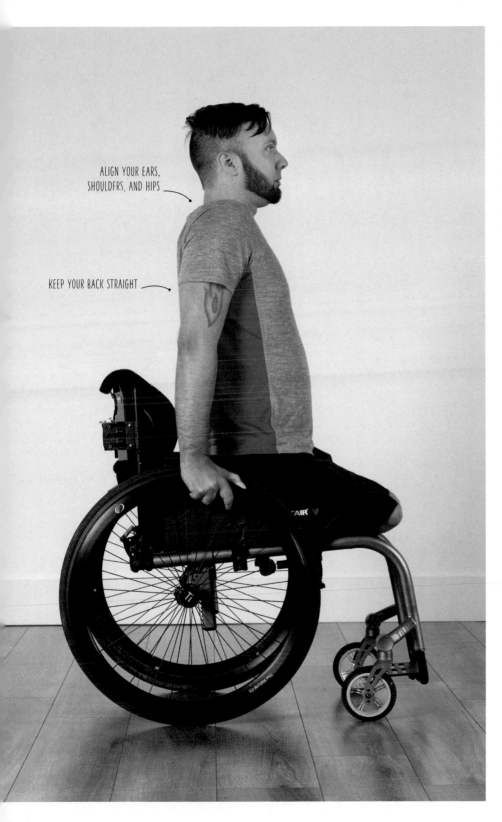

ALIGN YOUR EARS, SHOULDERS, AND HIPS

KEEP YOUR BACK STRAIGHT

<<< VARIATION #2

1. Sit in a chair, with your feet flat on the floor and your arms relaxed at your sides.
2. Press your hands into the sides of the chair and press down through your buttocks. Hold this position for 3 to 5 full breaths.

ALEX

WHO IS ALEXANDRA TRAUBERT?

I'm a combination of thought, expression, and long-left impressions. I'm continuously growing, experiencing, and learning about the world around me. I'm a soon-to-be mother, devoted wife, and loving daughter who was taught to be strong, caring, thoughtful, and passionate.

WHAT OBSERVATIONS HAVE YOU MADE ABOUT YOURSELF WHILE PRACTICING YOGA?

I've noticed the usual things people often have when performing yoga: being bent over in front of people, shaking and not maintaining my balance while holding poses, maybe not being flexible enough. But I've also noticed that I'm not the only one who has these kinds of issues. I love seeing people of every age (even over 80!), size, shape, etc., in yoga classes. It's an invigorating workout, and it helps me feel centered. I wouldn't say it's changed my life, but it's definitely a nice experience when my husband and I do it in the yard on a nice day or in a class with others.

WHAT WOULD YOU TELL OTHERS WHO MIGHT BE AFRAID TO TRY YOGA?

There's nothing to be afraid of—yoga is meant for any/everybody. I've been in classes with people of all kinds of shapes, ages, and capabilities that every pose is able to accommodate. Yoga is something that helps you be healthy, take your mind and body to the next level, connect with others on a spiritual level, and find that extra balance and inner peace. Yoga is a lifestyle.

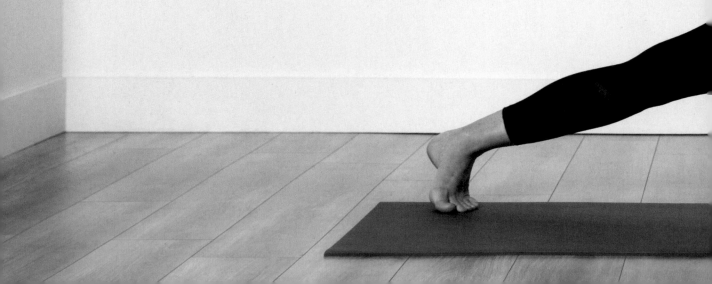

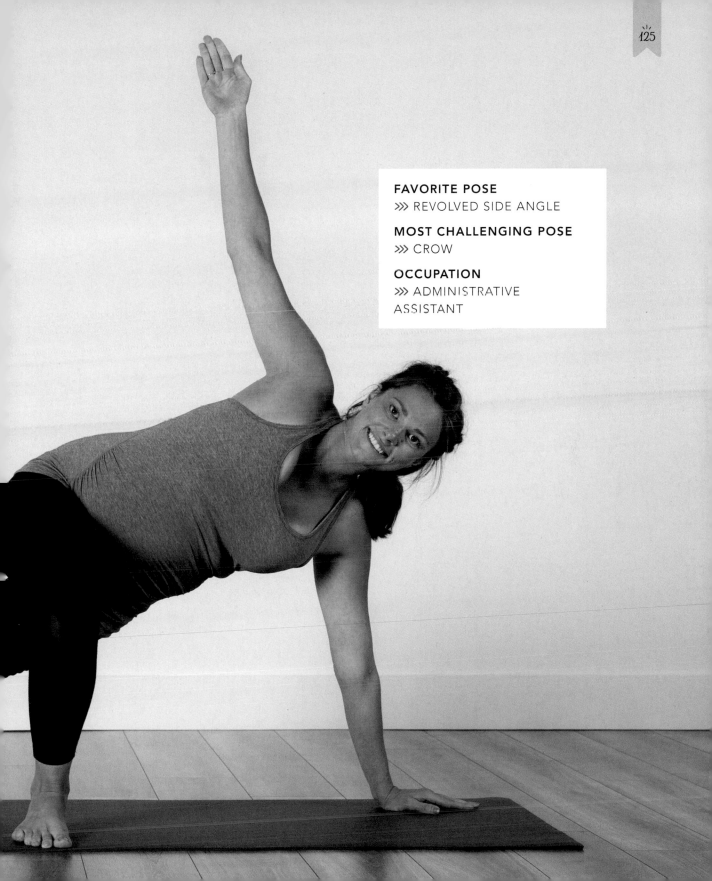

FAVORITE POSE
>>> REVOLVED SIDE ANGLE

MOST CHALLENGING POSE
>>> CROW

OCCUPATION
>>> ADMINISTRATIVE
ASSISTANT

Butterfly

>>> BADDHA KONASANA <<<

Spread your wings with this seated hip opener that also targets your groin muscles. Folding forward during this pose can also help ease lower-back pain. This is an especially great pose to perform during pregnancy.

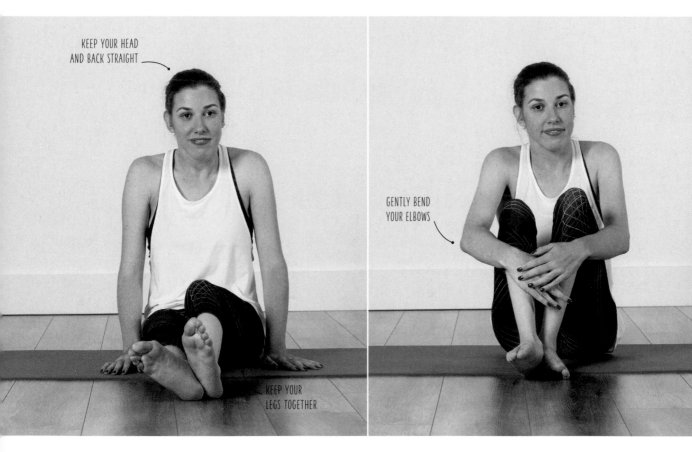

KEEP YOUR HEAD AND BACK STRAIGHT

GENTLY BEND YOUR ELBOWS

KEEP YOUR LEGS TOGETHER

1 Sit on the mat, with your legs extended and your arms relaxed at your sides. (You can also sit on a folded blanket.)

2 Bend your knees and bring your feet toward your sitting bones, placing your hands on your shins. (If you feel pain, pressure, or discomfort in your knees, place your feet farther away from your body.) Press the outer edges of your feet and your sitting bones into the mat.

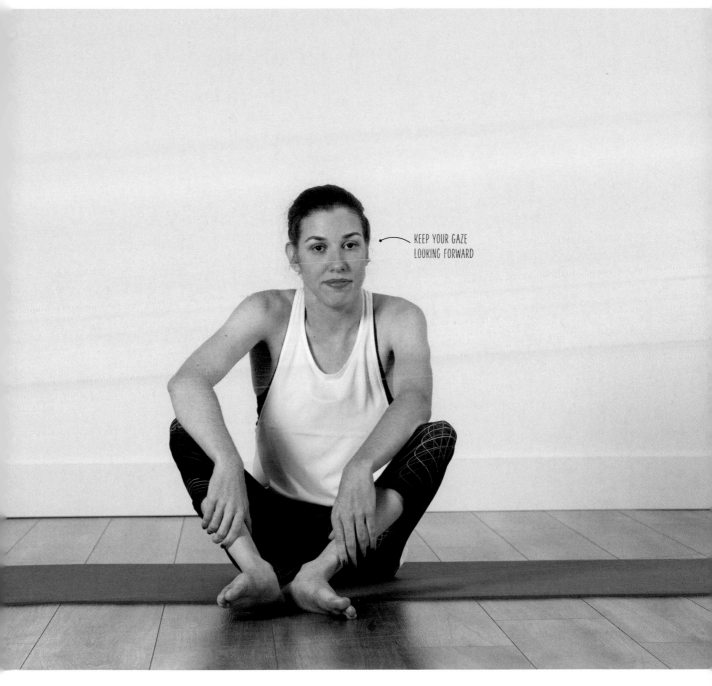

KEEP YOUR GAZE
LOOKING FORWARD

3 Push apart your legs. On an exhale, bend at your waist and lean forward and rest your inner forearms on the inside of your thighs. Hold this position for 3 to 5 full breaths.

～ BUTTERFLY ～
VARIATIONS

This pose comes with several variations, including using a prop to help with support. At least one of these can provide more comfort and stability for you.

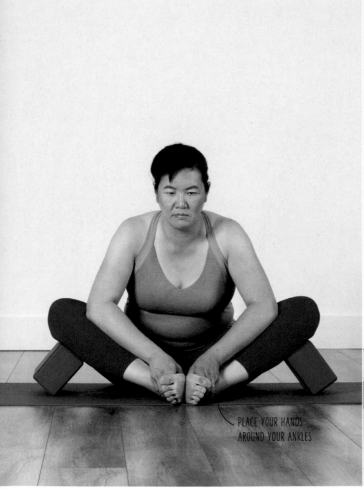

PLACE YOUR HANDS AROUND YOUR ANKLES

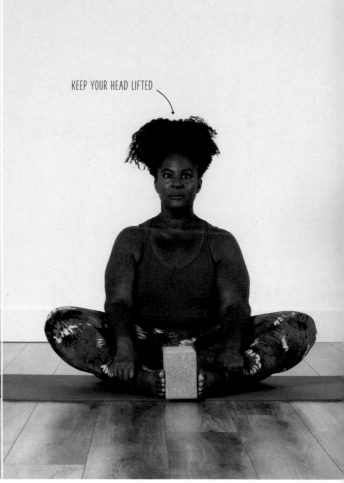

KEEP YOUR HEAD LIFTED

⫷⫷ VARIATION #1

Place a block near each leg. In step 3, place a knee on each block. (Adjust the height and placement as needed.)

⫷⫷ VARIATION #2

In step 3, place a block between the soles of your feet. (You can also create more of a diamond shape with your legs.)

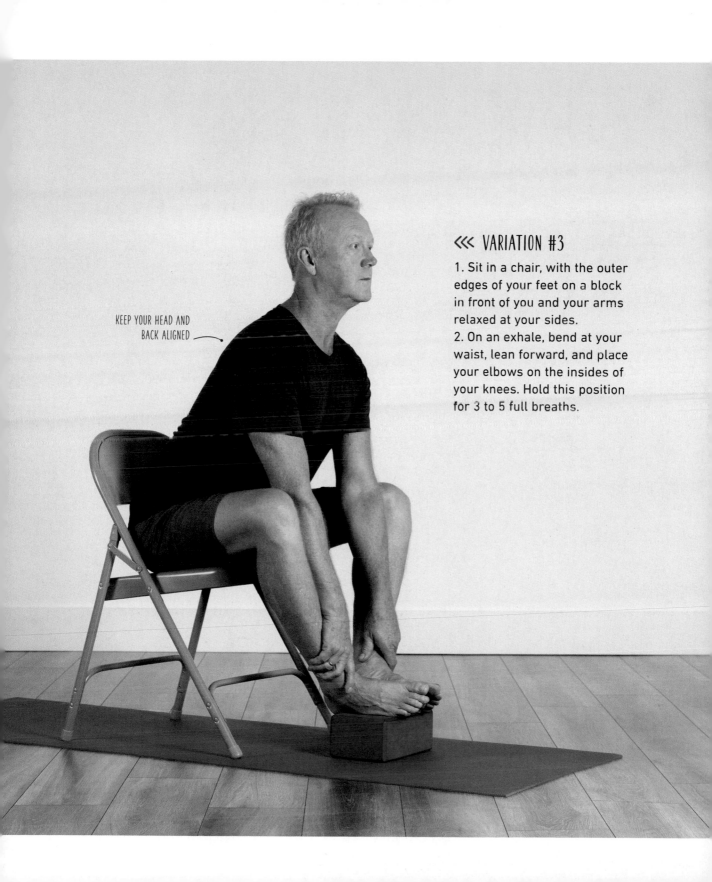

KEEP YOUR HEAD AND
BACK ALIGNED

⫷⫷⫷ VARIATION #3

1. Sit in a chair, with the outer edges of your feet on a block in front of you and your arms relaxed at your sides.

2. On an exhale, bend at your waist, lean forward, and place your elbows on the insides of your knees. Hold this position for 3 to 5 full breaths.

Pigeon

>>>EKA PADA RAJAKAPOTASANA<<<

This pose is a deep hip opener that can also help with lower-back pain, tight or sore hips, and overall well-being. Although these movements are challenging, you can benefit from the release of tension in your hips and back.

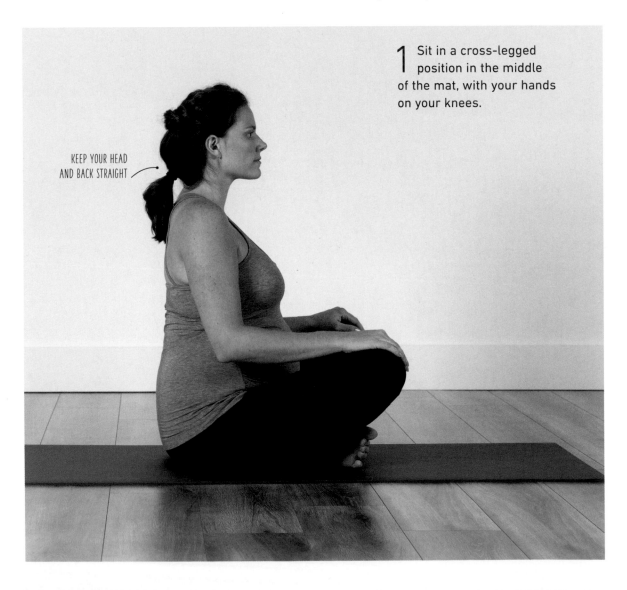

1 Sit in a cross-legged position in the middle of the mat, with your hands on your knees.

KEEP YOUR HEAD AND BACK STRAIGHT

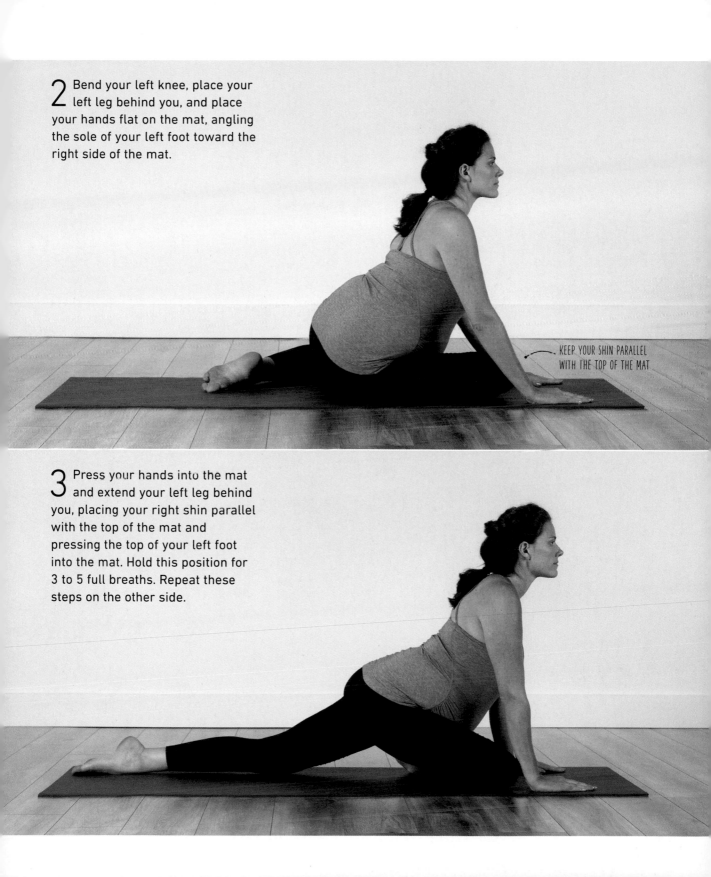

2 Bend your left knee, place your left leg behind you, and place your hands flat on the mat, angling the sole of your left foot toward the right side of the mat.

KEEP YOUR SHIN PARALLEL WITH THE TOP OF THE MAT

3 Press your hands into the mat and extend your left leg behind you, placing your right shin parallel with the top of the mat and pressing the top of your left foot into the mat. Hold this position for 3 to 5 full breaths. Repeat these steps on the other side.

‿ PIGEON ‿
VARIATIONS

If you decide you're not sure about this pose, try one of these accessible variations. You can still attain similar benefits to the main pose.

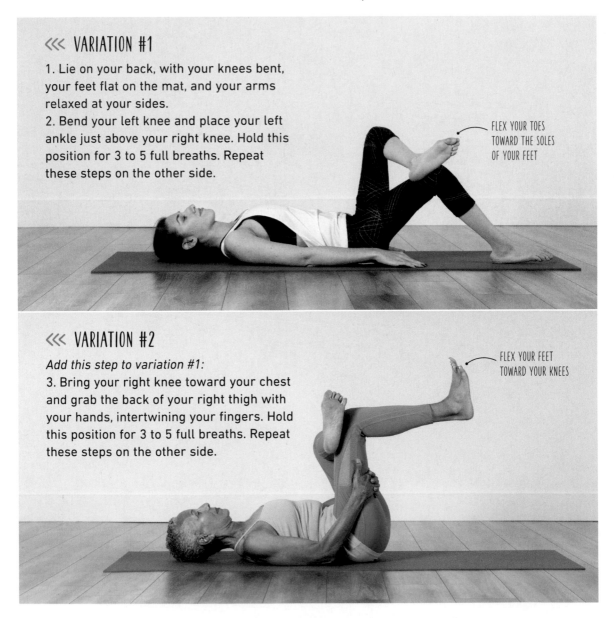

‹‹‹ VARIATION #1

1. Lie on your back, with your knees bent, your feet flat on the mat, and your arms relaxed at your sides.
2. Bend your left knee and place your left ankle just above your right knee. Hold this position for 3 to 5 full breaths. Repeat these steps on the other side.

FLEX YOUR TOES TOWARD THE SOLES OF YOUR FEET

‹‹‹ VARIATION #2

Add this step to variation #1:
3. Bring your right knee toward your chest and grab the back of your right thigh with your hands, intertwining your fingers. Hold this position for 3 to 5 full breaths. Repeat these steps on the other side.

FLEX YOUR FEET TOWARD YOUR KNEES

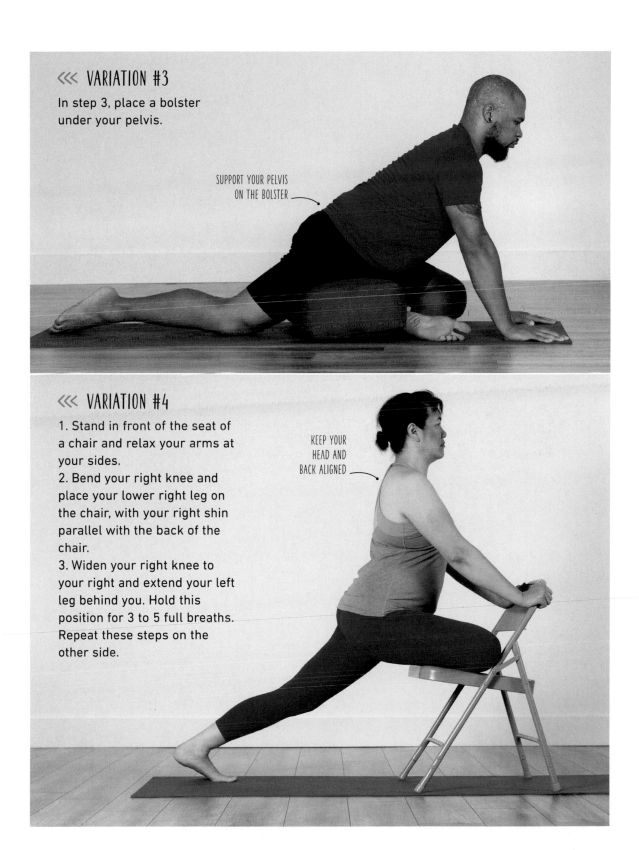

≪≪ VARIATION #3

In step 3, place a bolster under your pelvis.

SUPPORT YOUR PELVIS ON THE BOLSTER

≪≪ VARIATION #4

1. Stand in front of the seat of a chair and relax your arms at your sides.
2. Bend your right knee and place your lower right leg on the chair, with your right shin parallel with the back of the chair.
3. Widen your right knee to your right and extend your left leg behind you. Hold this position for 3 to 5 full breaths. Repeat these steps on the other side.

KEEP YOUR HEAD AND BACK ALIGNED

Eagle

>>> GARUDASANA <<<

You can soar like a majestic bird with this pose. It's excellent for developing and enhancing balance, strength, and flexibility throughout your body. This pose also helps you draw energy into the center of your body.

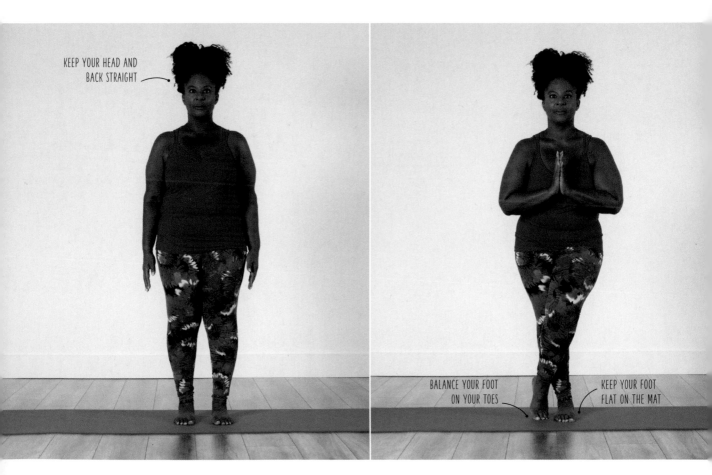

KEEP YOUR HEAD AND BACK STRAIGHT

BALANCE YOUR FOOT ON YOUR TOES

KEEP YOUR FOOT FLAT ON THE MAT

1 Stand in the middle of the mat, with your weight balanced equally between your feet and your arms relaxed at your sides.

2 Shift your weight to your right leg and bend your left knee. Bring your left leg across your right leg to align the back of your left knee with the front of your right knee. Place your hands in a prayer position in front of your chest.

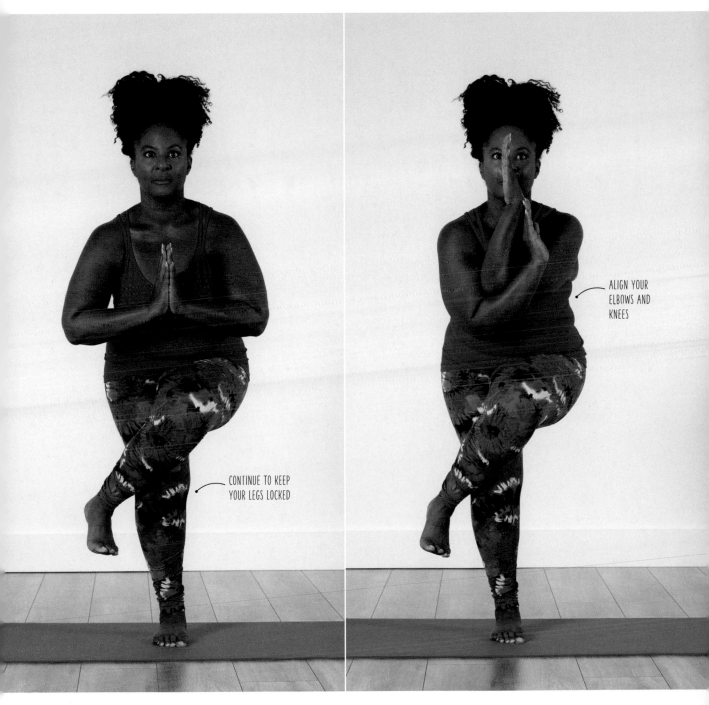

ALIGN YOUR
ELBOWS AND
KNEES

CONTINUE TO KEEP
YOUR LEGS LOCKED

3 Press your thighs together, slightly bend
your right knee, and shift your weight
backward as if lowering yourself into a chair.

4 Hook your right arm under your left elbow
until your elbows align. (Or cross your right
elbow with your left triceps.) Hold this position
for 3 to 5 full breaths. Repeat these steps on the
other side.

～EAGLE～
VARIATIONS

Using props, like blocks, a wall, and the mat, can help make this pose more accessible—if not a little easier. And don't worry—you can still fly with all the other eagles.

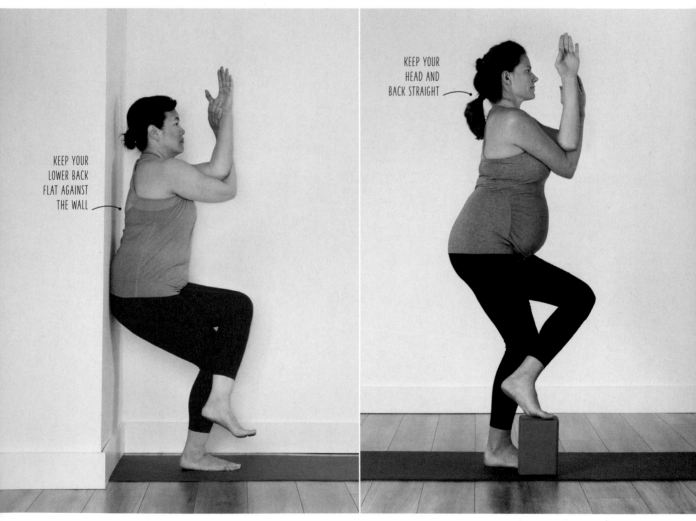

KEEP YOUR LOWER BACK FLAT AGAINST THE WALL

KEEP YOUR HEAD AND BACK STRAIGHT

⟪⟪ VARIATION #1

In step 1, stand facing away from a wall. In step 2, press your back into the wall when crossing your legs.

⟪⟪ VARIATION #2

Place a block short edge up on the outside of your right leg. In step 2, place your left foot on the block.

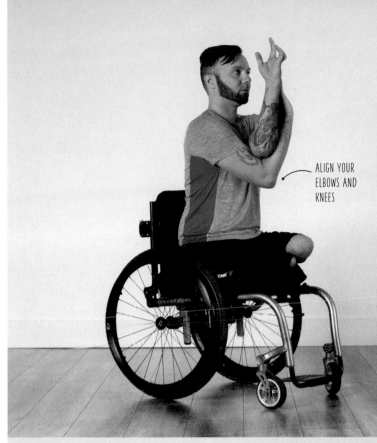

ALIGN YOUR
ELBOWS AND
KNEES

⟨⟨⟨ VARIATION #3

1. Sit on the edge of a chair, with your arms relaxed at your sides.
2. Bend your left knee and cross your left leg over your right thigh.
3. Hook your right arm under your left elbow until your elbows align. Hold this position for 3 to 5 full breaths. Repeat these steps on the other side.

⟨⟨⟨ VARIATION #4

1. Lie on your back, with your arms relaxed at your sides.
2. Bend your right knee and cross your right leg over your left thigh.
3. Bend your elbows and hook your right arm under your left elbow until your elbows align. Hold this position for 3 to 5 full breaths. Repeat these steps on the other side.

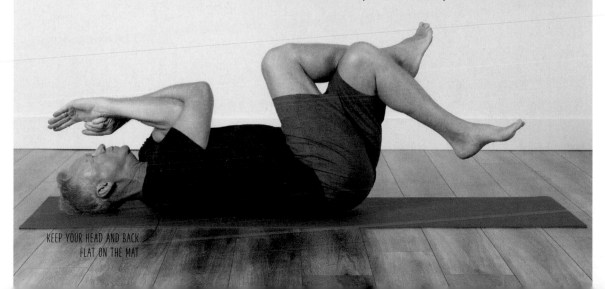

KEEP YOUR HEAD AND BACK
FLAT ON THE MAT

Crow

>>> KAKASANA <<<

Arm balancing is a great way to build upper-body strength while also testing your fortitude. This pose demands core strength, which you will also develop. What's unusual about this pose is that your knees rest on the backs of your arms.

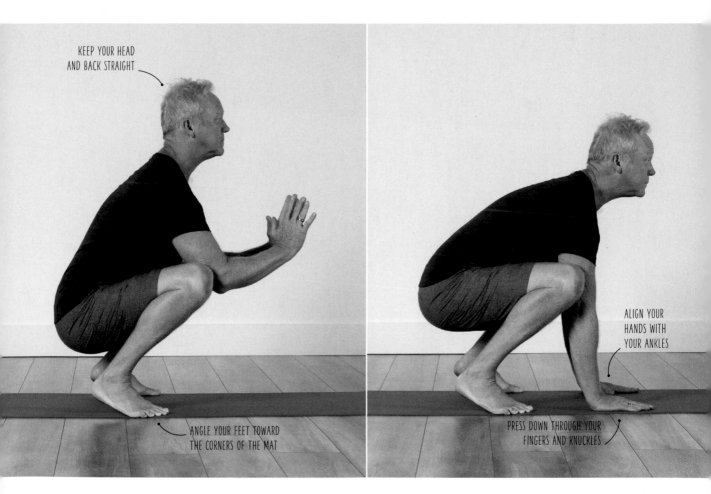

KEEP YOUR HEAD AND BACK STRAIGHT

ANGLE YOUR FEET TOWARD THE CORNERS OF THE MAT

ALIGN YOUR HANDS WITH YOUR ANKLES

PRESS DOWN THROUGH YOUR FINGERS AND KNUCKLES

1 Squat in the middle of the mat, with your elbows resting on the inside of your knees, your heels lifted off the mat, and your hands in a prayer position in front of your chest.

2 Place your hands flat on the mat in front of you and press your elbows into the sides of your knees.

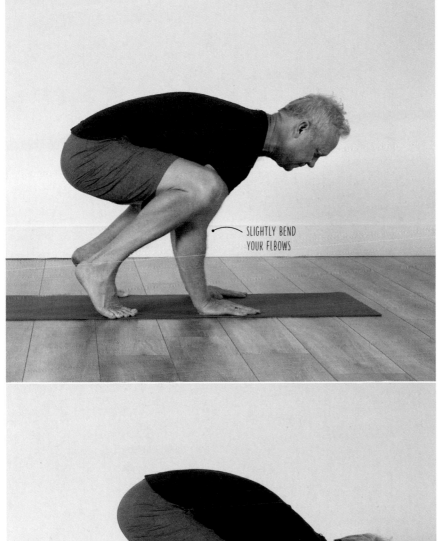

SLIGHTLY BEND YOUR ELBOWS

3 Gently lean forward, pressing your hands into the mat and gazing at the top of the mat.

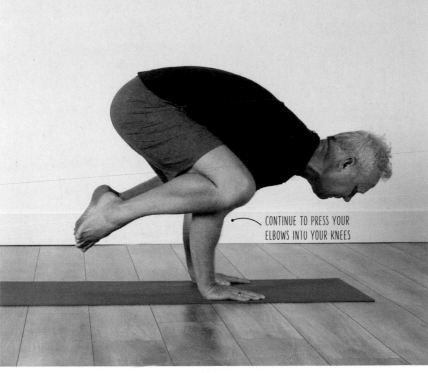

CONTINUE TO PRESS YOUR ELBOWS INTO YOUR KNEES

4 Press down through the ball of your right foot to lift your right leg off the mat. When you find your balance, press down through the ball of your left foot to lift your left leg off the mat. Hold this position for 3 to 5 full breaths.

∾ CROW ∾
VARIATIONS

Our fear of falling often stops us from taking flight.
These variations can help ease some of your concerns
as you allow yourself to experience the sensation of flying.

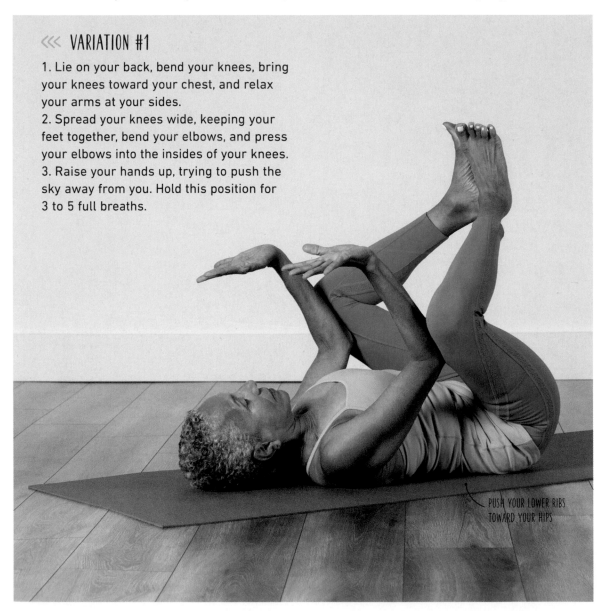

⟪ VARIATION #1

1. Lie on your back, bend your knees, bring your knees toward your chest, and relax your arms at your sides.
2. Spread your knees wide, keeping your feet together, bend your elbows, and press your elbows into the insides of your knees.
3. Raise your hands up, trying to push the sky away from you. Hold this position for 3 to 5 full breaths.

PUSH YOUR LOWER RIBS
TOWARD YOUR HIPS

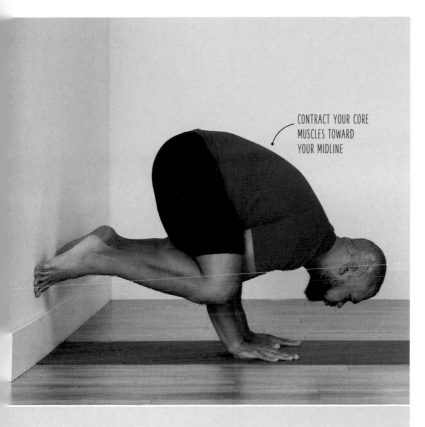

CONTRACT YOUR CORE MUSCLES TOWARD YOUR MIDLINE

⫷ VARIATION #2

1. Stand facing away from a wall, with your weight balanced equally between your feet and your arms relaxed at your sides.

2. Bend your knees, lift your heels off the mat, and slowly lower yourself into a squat. Place your elbows on the inside of your knees and place your hands flat on the mat in front of you.

3. Gently lean forward, pressing more weight into your hands, walk your feet up the wall, and place your toes against the wall. Use your arms to push the mat away from you. Hold this position for 3 to 5 full breaths.

⫷ VARIATION #3

1. Sit on the edge of a chair, with your feet on the legs of the chair and your arms relaxed at your sides.

2. Bend at your waist, lean forward to place your hands flat on the floor, and slide your feet up the legs of the chair. (You can also place your hands on blocks.) Hold this position for 3 to 5 full breaths.

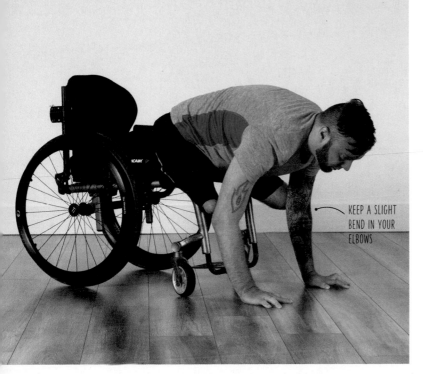

KEEP A SLIGHT BEND IN YOUR ELBOWS

Warrior 1

>>>VIRABHADRASANA 1<<<

This is an excellent pose for creating strength and power in your legs. It's part of the Warrior series of yoga poses, which can help build stability in your body—and make you feel like nothing can stop you.

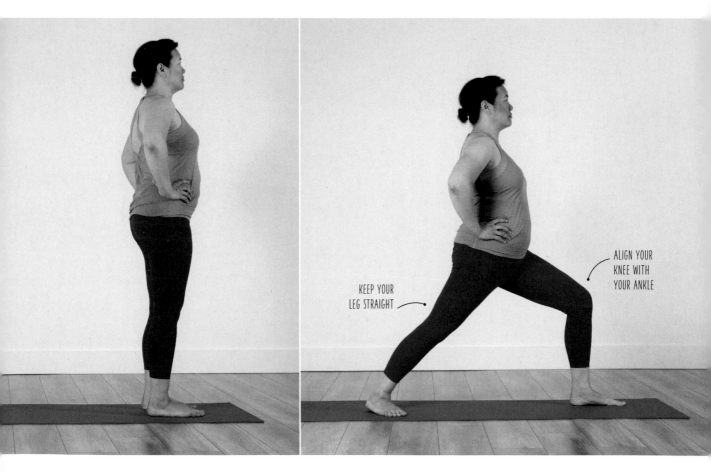

KEEP YOUR LEG STRAIGHT

ALIGN YOUR KNEE WITH YOUR ANKLE

1 Stand at the top of the mat, with your weight balanced equally between your feet and your hands on your hips.

2 Extend your right leg behind you, with your toes angled toward the top-right corner of the mat and your upper body parallel with the top of the mat, and slightly bend your left knee. (If you can't see the toes of your left foot, widen your stance by spreading your legs farther apart.)

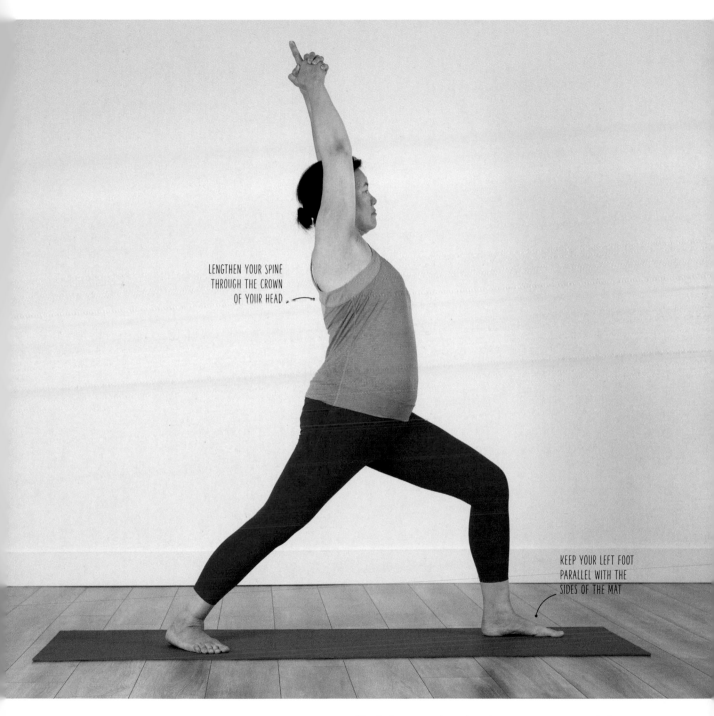

LENGTHEN YOUR SPINE THROUGH THE CROWN OF YOUR HEAD

KEEP YOUR LEFT FOOT PARALLEL WITH THE SIDES OF THE MAT

3 Raise your head and your arms toward the sky, with your hands in a prayer position over your head. Hold this position for 3 to 5 full breaths. Repeat these steps on the other side.

∽ WARRIOR 1 ∽
VARIATIONS

This pose requires strength and balance in your legs, but using the mat or a chair can help you build strength and balance—and make these movements more accessible.

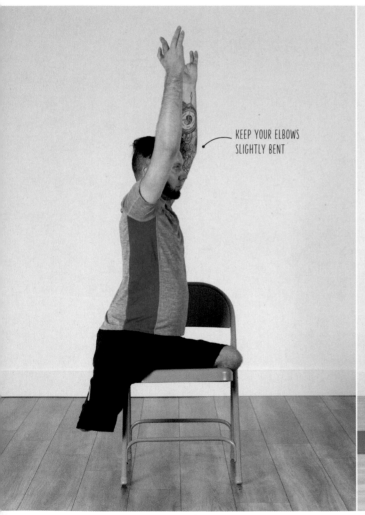

KEEP YOUR ELBOWS SLIGHTLY BENT

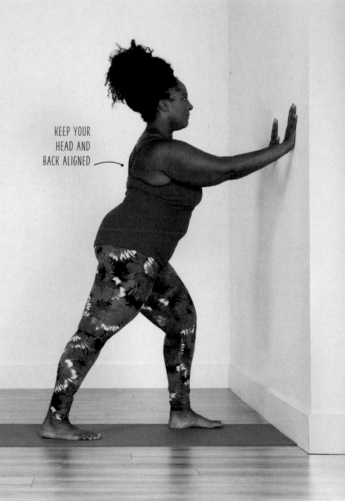

KEEP YOUR HEAD AND BACK ALIGNED

≪ VARIATION #1

In step 2, place your left thigh across the seat of a chair before stepping your right leg behind you.

≪ VARIATION #2

In step 1, stand facing a wall. In step 2, place your hands flat on the wall and bend your left knee.

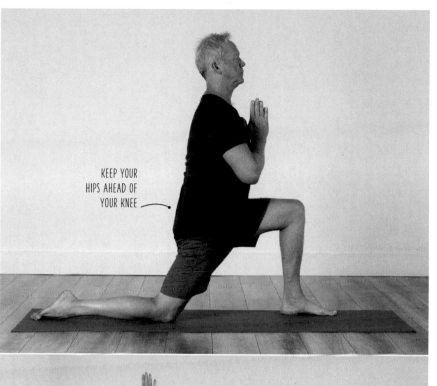

KEEP YOUR
HIPS AHEAD OF
YOUR KNEE

«« VARIATION #3

In step 2, place your
right knee on the mat.

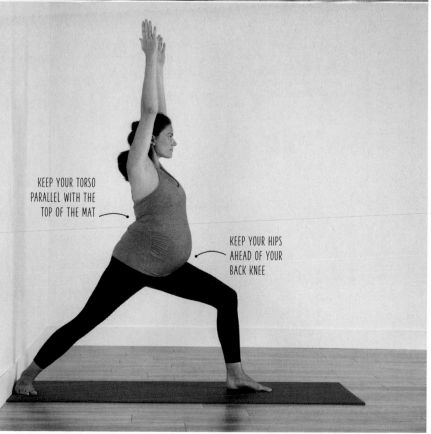

KEEP YOUR TORSO
PARALLEL WITH THE
TOP OF THE MAT

KEEP YOUR HIPS
AHEAD OF YOUR
BACK KNEE

«« VARIATION #4

1. Place the short
edge of a mat
perpendicular to
a wall. Stand facing
a few feet away from
the wall.
2. Extend your right
leg behind you and
place the outer edge
of your right foot
against the wall.
3. Raise your arms
toward the sky,
facing your palms
toward each other.
Hold this position for
3 to 5 full breaths.
Repeat these steps on
the other side.

Warrior 2

>>> VIRABHADRASANA 2 <<<

Movements in this strong standing pose are excellent for building strength in your legs, lengthening your spine, and opening your chest, shoulders, hips, and arms. This added power can help you be an amazing everyday warrior.

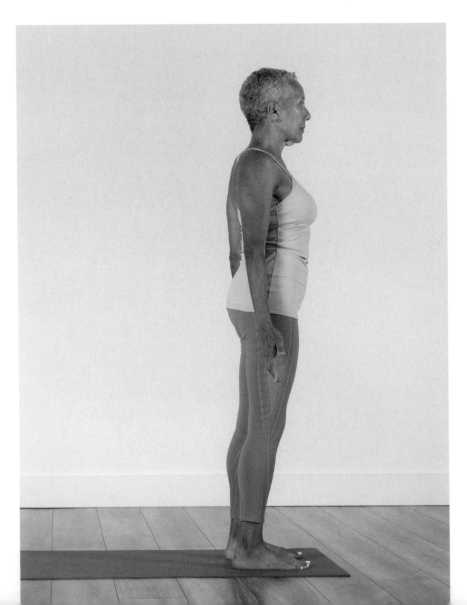

1 Stand at the top of the mat, with your weight balanced equally between your feet, your palms facing forward, your shoulder blades pulled together, and your arms relaxed at your sides.

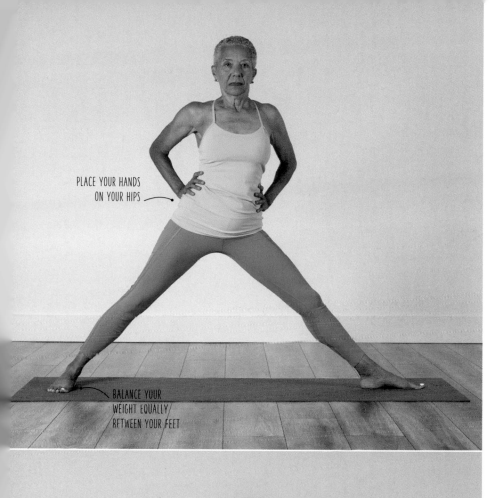

PLACE YOUR HANDS
ON YOUR HIPS

BALANCE YOUR
WEIGHT EQUALLY
BETWEEN YOUR FEET

2 Extend your right leg behind you and turn your right foot until parallel with the back of the mat. Make sure you can see the toes of your left foot. (If you can't, widen your stance by stepping your legs farther apart.)

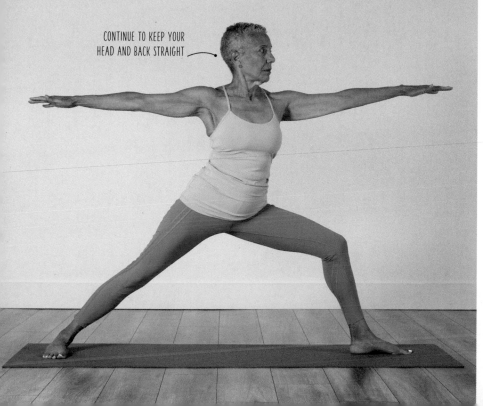

CONTINUE TO KEEP YOUR
HEAD AND BACK STRAIGHT

3 Push your legs apart energetically and bend deeply with your left knee. Raise your arms to form a T, lengthen your spine through the crown of your head, and gaze over your left arm. Hold this position for 3 to 5 full breaths. Repeat these steps on the other side.

~ WARRIOR 2 ~

VARIATIONS

This pose is all about strength and balance in your legs.
To help build and enhance those, you can perform
this pose using the mat, a chair, or a wall.

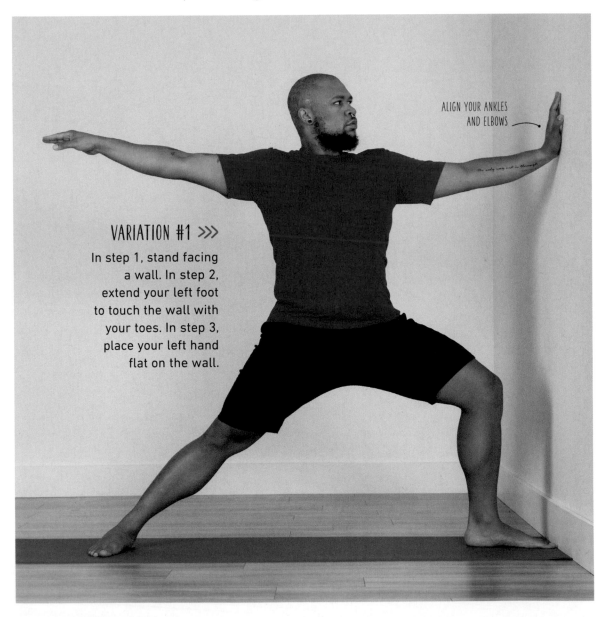

ALIGN YOUR ANKLES
AND ELBOWS

VARIATION #1 >>>

In step 1, stand facing
a wall. In step 2,
extend your left foot
to touch the wall with
your toes. In step 3,
place your left hand
flat on the wall.

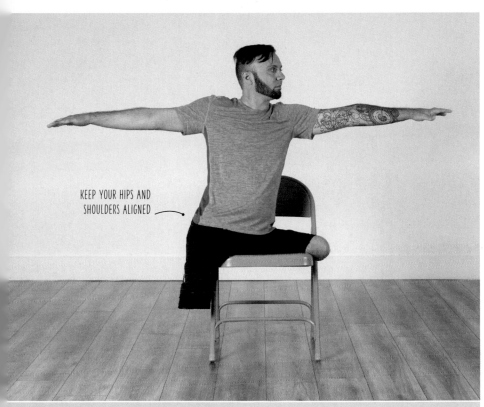

KEEP YOUR HIPS AND SHOULDERS ALIGNED

‹‹‹ VARIATION #2

1. Sit in a chair, with your feet flat on the floor and your arms relaxed at your sides.
2. Rotate your body to your right, extend your right leg behind you, and place your left thigh across the seat of the chair.
3. Extend your arms to form a T. Hold this position for 3 to 5 full breaths. Repeat these steps on the other side.

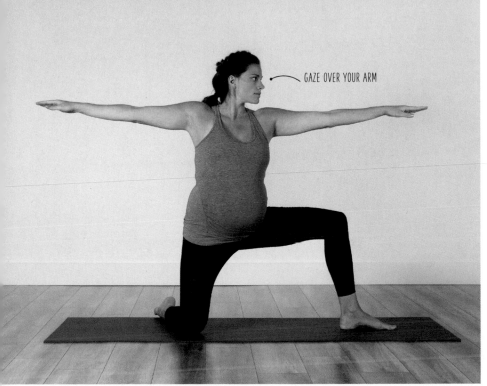

GAZE OVER YOUR ARM

‹‹‹ VARIATION #3

In step 2, place your right knee on the mat and rotate your right hip until your lower-right leg is parallel with the back of the mat.

Warrior 3

>>> VIRABHADRASANA 3 <<<

This is sometimes referred to as Airplane pose because it makes you feel like you're gliding through the air. These movements are excellent for building balance, learning how to focus on your breath, and creating strength in your legs.

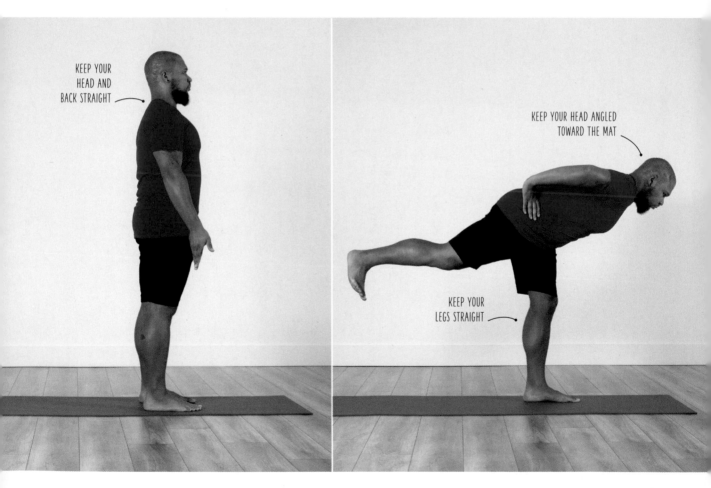

KEEP YOUR HEAD AND BACK STRAIGHT

KEEP YOUR HEAD ANGLED TOWARD THE MAT

KEEP YOUR LEGS STRAIGHT

1 Stand at the top of the mat, with your weight balanced equally between your feet and your arms relaxed at your sides, facing your palms forward.

2 On an exhale, bend at your waist and place your hands on your hips. Extend your right leg behind you until your upper body and right leg are parallel with the mat.

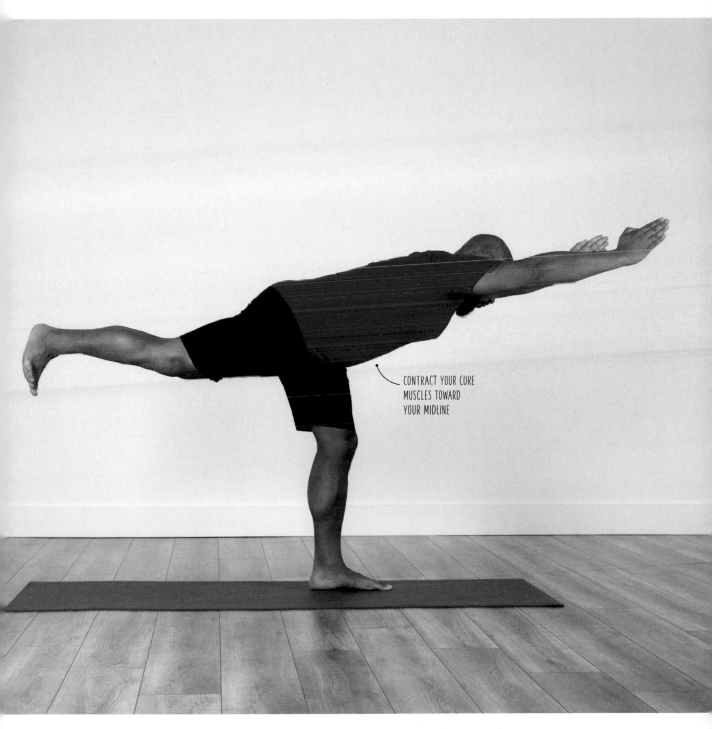

CONTRACT YOUR CORE
MUSCLES TOWARD
YOUR MIDLINE

3 Once you find your balance, extend your arms until parallel with the mat. Hold this position for 3 to 5 full breaths. Repeat these steps on the other side.

~ WARRIOR 3 ~
# VARIATIONS

Taking flight into this pose can prove somewhat challenging, but using a chair or a wall can help make this pose more accessible and more balanced.

⟪ VARIATION #1

In step 1, stand between two chairs, with their seats facing you. In step 2, place your right leg over the back of the chair behind you. In step 3, place your arms across the back of the chair in front of you. (You can also place your arms across the chair in front of you before extending your right leg across the chair behind you.)

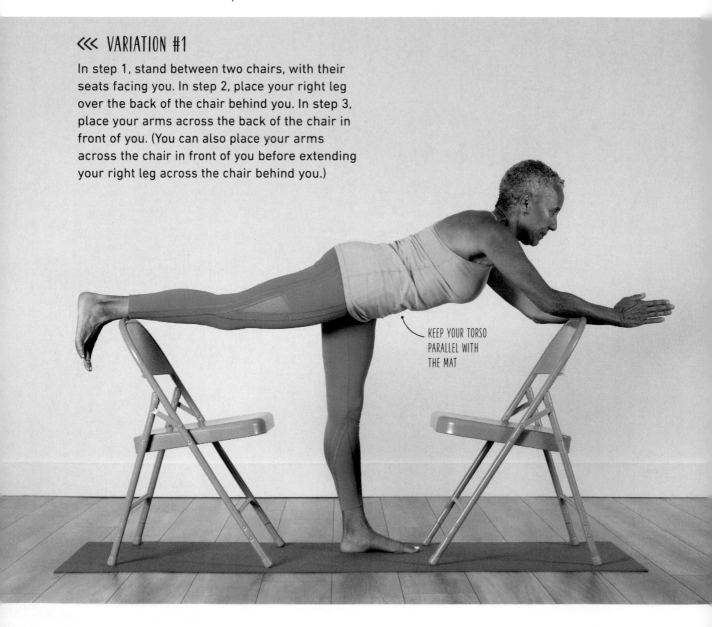

KEEP YOUR TORSO PARALLEL WITH THE MAT

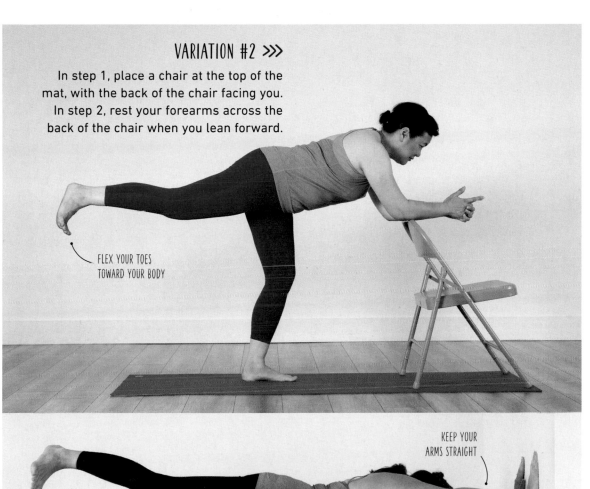

VARIATION #2 >>>

In step 1, place a chair at the top of the mat, with the back of the chair facing you. In step 2, rest your forearms across the back of the chair when you lean forward.

FLEX YOUR TOES
TOWARD YOUR BODY

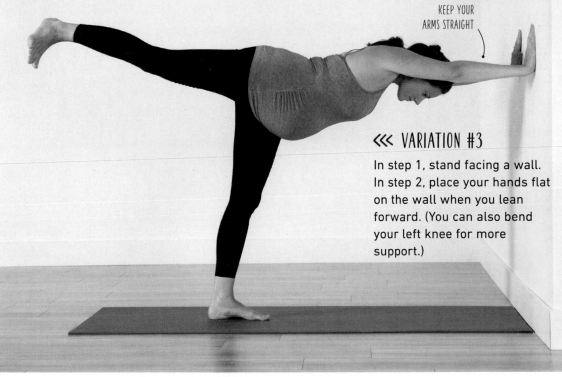

KEEP YOUR
ARMS STRAIGHT

<<< VARIATION #3

In step 1, stand facing a wall. In step 2, place your hands flat on the wall when you lean forward. (You can also bend your left knee for more support.)

Corpse

>>> SAVASANA <<<

This might seems easy, but it's one of the hardest poses to master. Because it involves the challenge of finding a deep state of relaxation—with the intention of letting go— this pose is one of the main reasons people practice yoga.

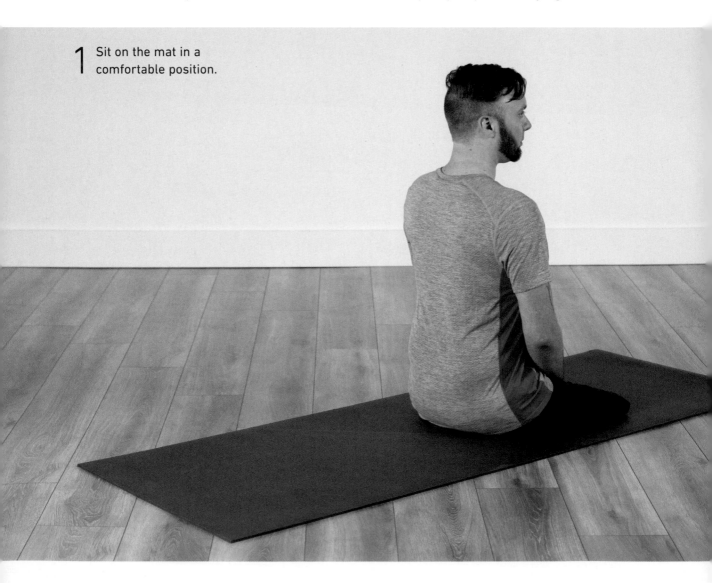

1 Sit on the mat in a comfortable position.

2 Lie on your back, rest your hands on your chest, and extend your legs. Relax every part of your body and feel yourself being supported by the mat beneath you. Observe your body from head to toe, surrendering to the present moment. Notice all the places where your body makes contact with the mat and release any tension in your muscles. With each exhalation, imagine your body getting heavier and sinking deeper into the mat. Release everything into the floor. Stay in this position for as long as desired.

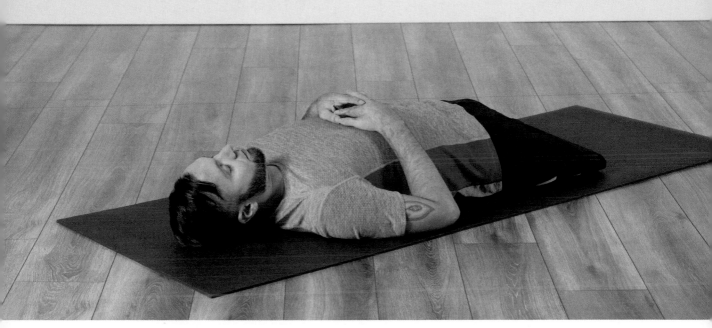

～CORPSE～
VARIATIONS

Lying flat on your back on a hard surface can sometimes feel uncomfortable. It's especially challenging if you have rounder buttocks or a curvy and inflexible lower back. These variations can make this pose more relaxing.

≪ VARIATION #1

In step 2, place your legs on top of an exercise ball.

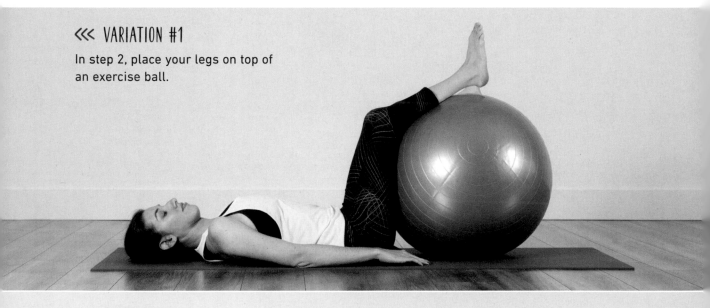

≪ VARIATION #2

In step 2, lie on your side and place a bolster between your legs.

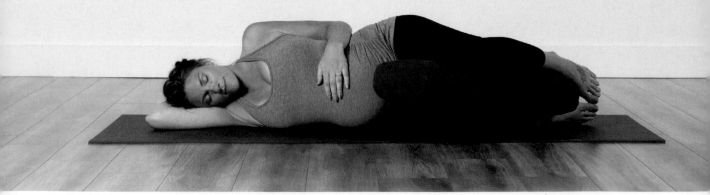

≪≪ VARIATION #3

In step 2, place your legs on
a chair or against a wall in
any comfortable position.

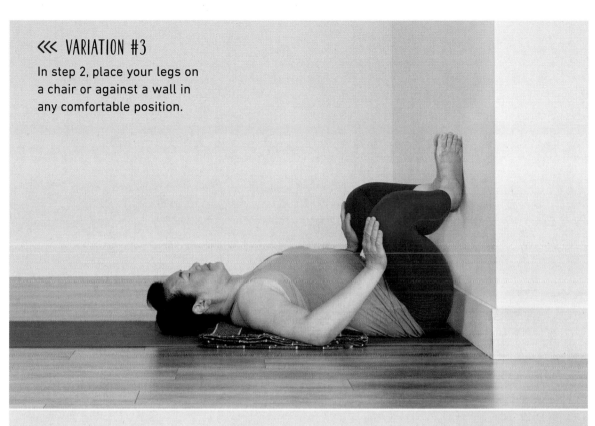

≪≪ VARIATION #4

In step 2, bend your knees and walk your
feet toward the sides of the mat. Keep the
soles of your feet flat against the mat and
let your knees fall toward each other,
allowing your knees to gently touch without
narrowing the distance between your
thighs. Extend your arms to form a T.
Release any muscle tension.

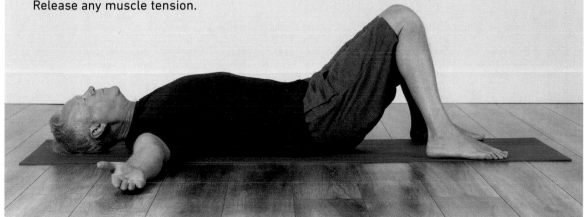

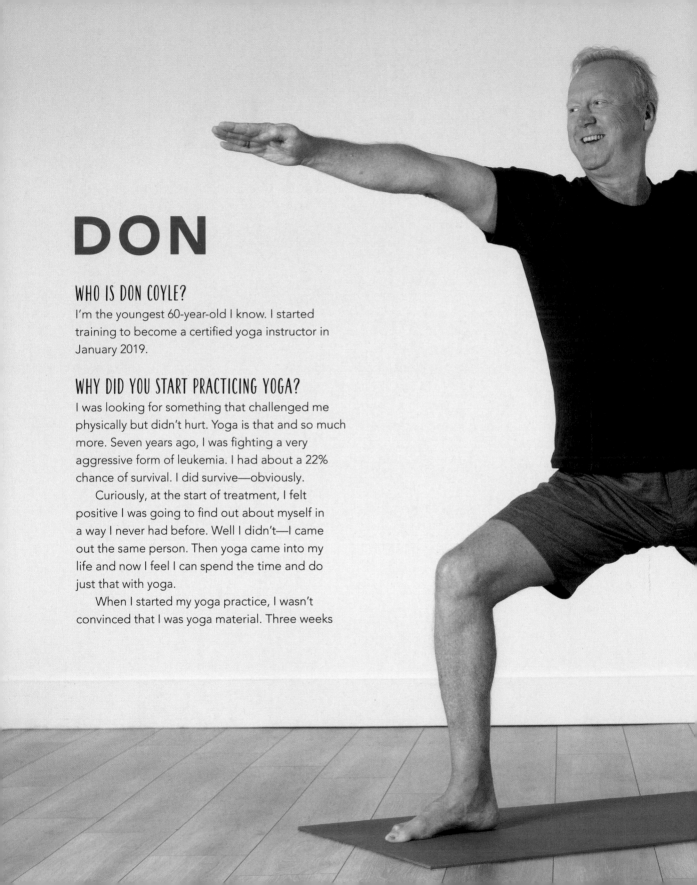

DON

WHO IS DON COYLE?

I'm the youngest 60-year-old I know. I started training to become a certified yoga instructor in January 2019.

WHY DID YOU START PRACTICING YOGA?

I was looking for something that challenged me physically but didn't hurt. Yoga is that and so much more. Seven years ago, I was fighting a very aggressive form of leukemia. I had about a 22% chance of survival. I did survive—obviously.

Curiously, at the start of treatment, I felt positive I was going to find out about myself in a way I never had before. Well I didn't—I came out the same person. Then yoga came into my life and now I feel I can spend the time and do just that with yoga.

When I started my yoga practice, I wasn't convinced that I was yoga material. Three weeks

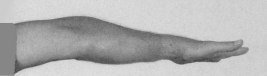

FAVORITE POSE
>>> WARRIOR 2

MOST CHALLENGING POSE
>>> CROW

OCCUPATION
>>> DESIGNING PRODUCTION
TOOLS FOR THE AUTO
INDUSTRY

into it, I thought I had found something, but I still wasn't sure. It wasn't until I fully grasped the power of the meditative practice inside yoga that it clicked. I could find quiet in my life. I could shut out the madness of my day-to-day life and just breathe.

WHAT DO YOU ENJOY MOST ABOUT PRACTICING YOGA?

Yoga has built my strength, added power to my body, and made me way more physically prepared to face my particular journey. After a few months of practice, I felt more emotionally prepared. I feel better about my entire being because of this experience. Dianne is a big part of this. Her approach to yoga is the power I get from it. You can be afraid of yoga. I'm sure there are many different experiences in life that made you afraid. This is the one time you'll come out the other side—free and enlightened.

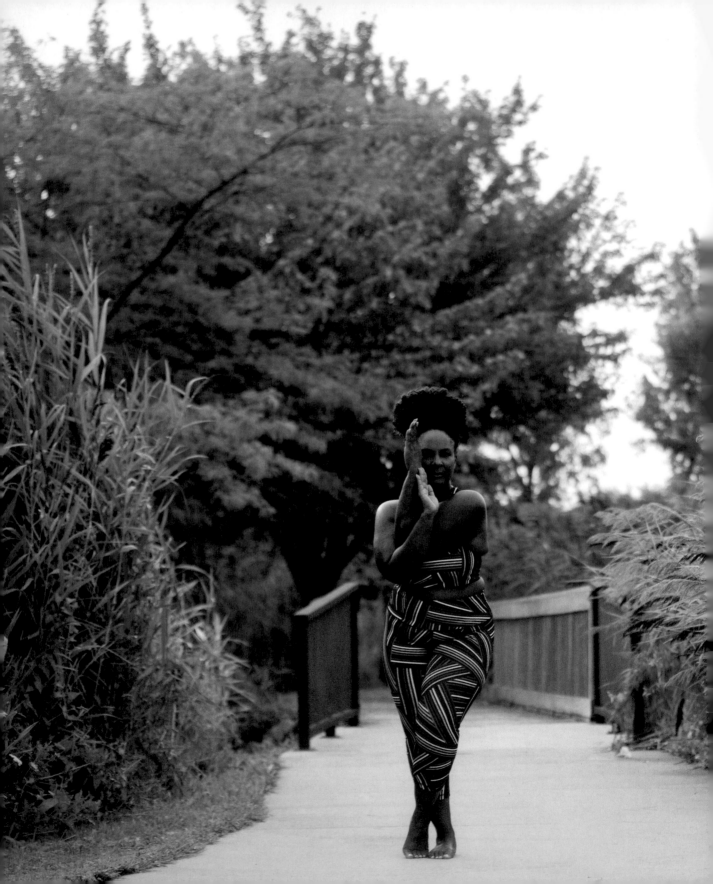

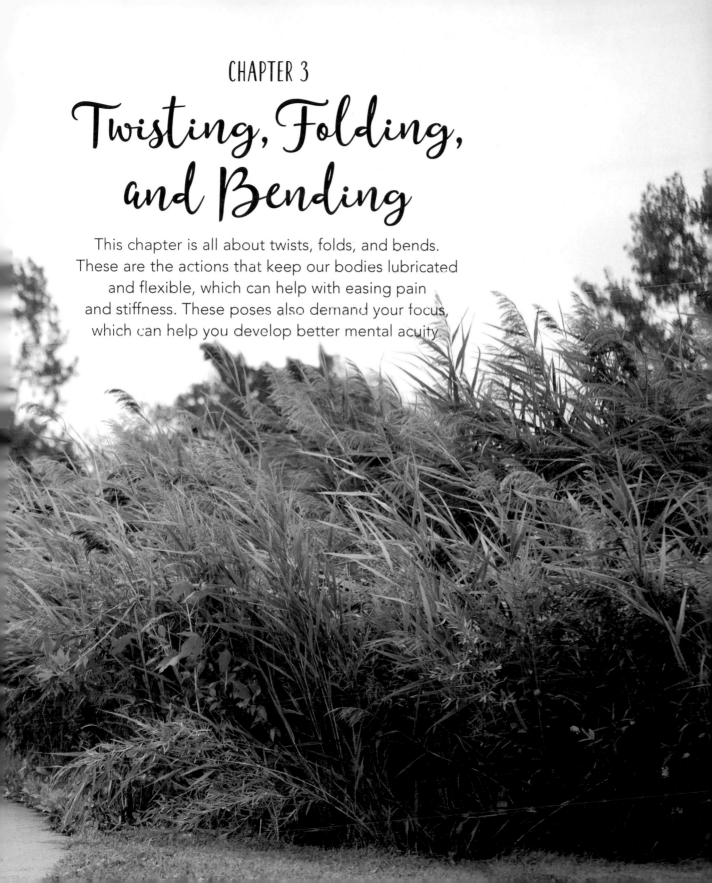

CHAPTER 3
Twisting, Folding, and Bending

This chapter is all about twists, folds, and bends.
These are the actions that keep our bodies lubricated
and flexible, which can help with easing pain
and stiffness. These poses also demand your focus,
which can help you develop better mental acuity.

Downward Dog

>>> ADHO MUKHA SVANASANA <<<

When you think about yoga, this pose is probably what first comes to mind. It can create length in muscles throughout your body, particularly your calves, hamstrings, glutes, hips, and lower back, and it can create upper-body strength.

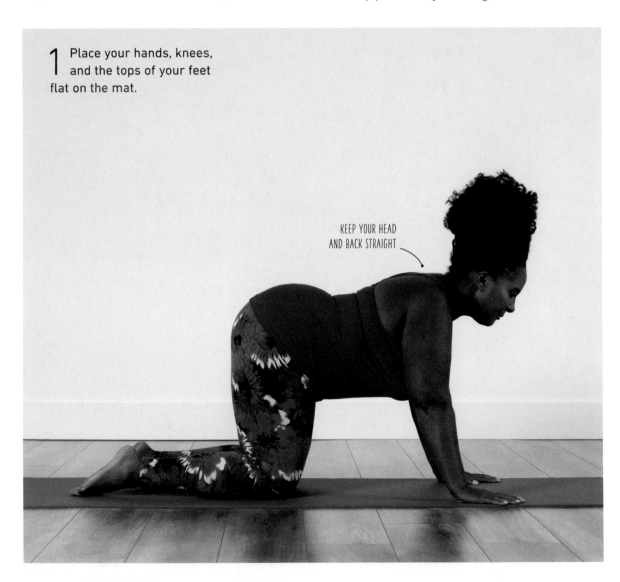

1 Place your hands, knees, and the tops of your feet flat on the mat.

KEEP YOUR HEAD AND BACK STRAIGHT

2 Walk your hands to just ahead of your shoulders and as wide as the mat. Press your fingers into the mat, engaging your index fingers and thumbs by pressing them deeper into the mat.

ALIGN YOUR OUTER SHOULDER WITH THE CENTER OF YOUR WRIST

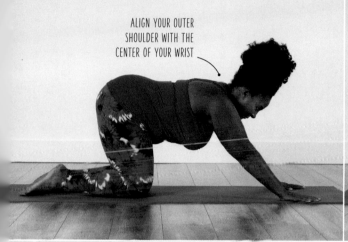

3 Curl your toes under and lift your hips up and back to form an inverted V. (If your hamstrings feel tight, keep your knees bent and the gluteal fold—where your legs meet your buttocks—lifted up.)

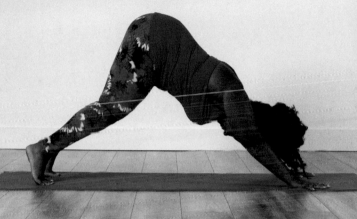

CONTINUE TO PUSH YOUR HIPS UP AND BACK

4 Pull your upper arms and triceps toward your ears, and use your upper arm strength to push the mat away from you. Hold this position for 3 to 5 full breaths.

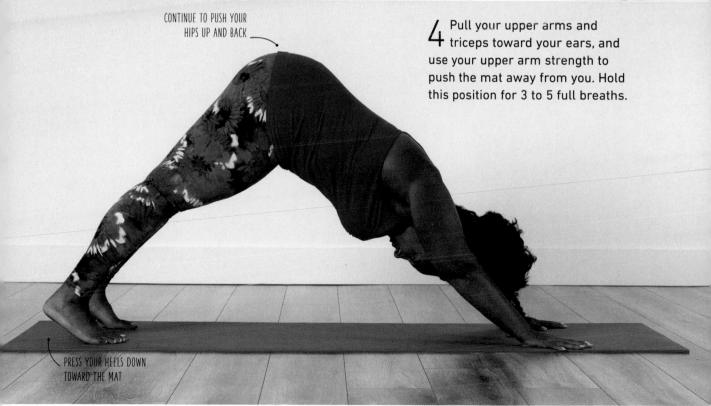

PRESS YOUR HEELS DOWN TOWARD THE MAT

∽ DOWNWARD DOG ∽
VARIATIONS

This pose can put pressure on your wrists and lower body.
These variations ease the physical stress while still allowing
you to extend your spine, engage your arms, and open your
shoulders and your upper-middle back.

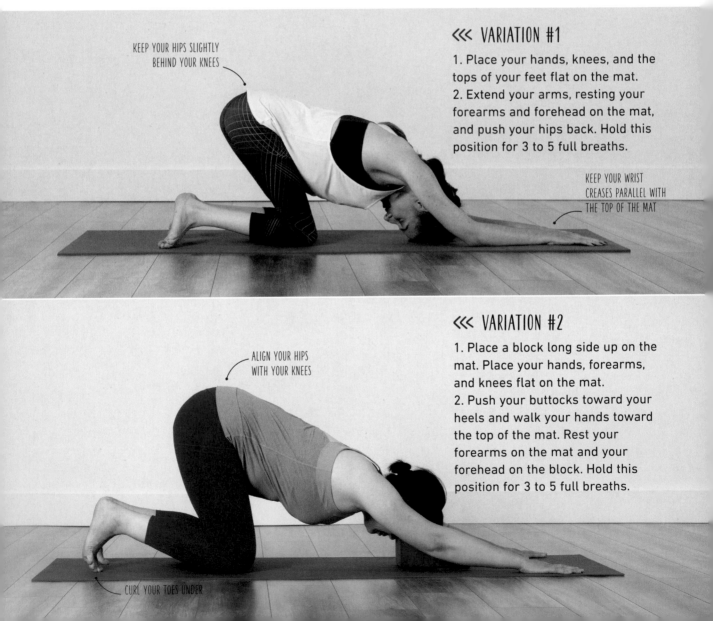

**KEEP YOUR HIPS SLIGHTLY
BEHIND YOUR KNEES**

**KEEP YOUR WRIST
CREASES PARALLEL WITH
THE TOP OF THE MAT**

≪ VARIATION #1

1. Place your hands, knees, and the
tops of your feet flat on the mat.
2. Extend your arms, resting your
forearms and forehead on the mat,
and push your hips back. Hold this
position for 3 to 5 full breaths.

**ALIGN YOUR HIPS
WITH YOUR KNEES**

CURL YOUR TOES UNDER

≪ VARIATION #2

1. Place a block long side up on the
mat. Place your hands, forearms,
and knees flat on the mat.
2. Push your buttocks toward your
heels and walk your hands toward
the top of the mat. Rest your
forearms on the mat and your
forehead on the block. Hold this
position for 3 to 5 full breaths.

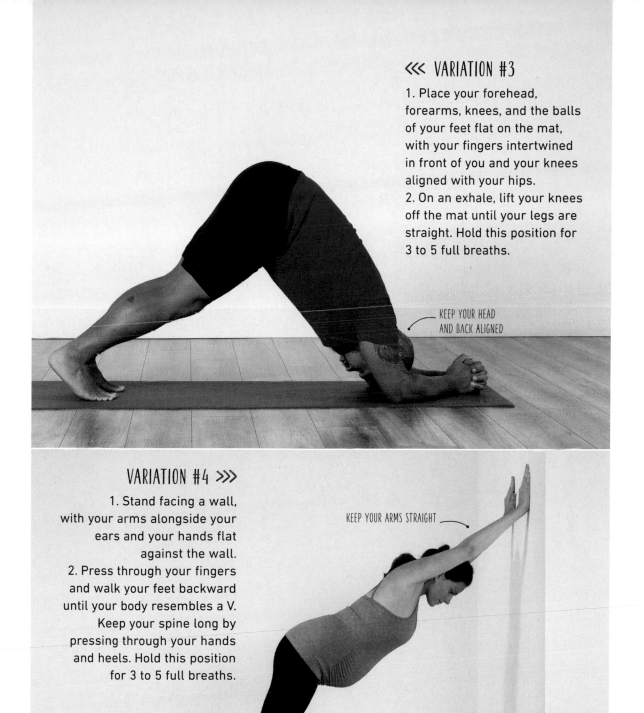

<<< VARIATION #3
1. Place your forehead, forearms, knees, and the balls of your feet flat on the mat, with your fingers intertwined in front of you and your knees aligned with your hips.
2. On an exhale, lift your knees off the mat until your legs are straight. Hold this position for 3 to 5 full breaths.

KEEP YOUR HEAD AND BACK ALIGNED

VARIATION #4 >>>
1. Stand facing a wall, with your arms alongside your ears and your hands flat against the wall.
2. Press through your fingers and walk your feet backward until your body resembles a V. Keep your spine long by pressing through your hands and heels. Hold this position for 3 to 5 full breaths.

KEEP YOUR ARMS STRAIGHT

Cobra

>>> BHUJANGASANA <<<

This is a popular backbending and heart-opening pose. Practicing these movements can open your shoulders, lengthen the muscles of the front of your body, and strengthen the muscles of your back and upper body.

1 Lie on your belly, with your arms folded under your head and your chin resting on your forearms, and extend your legs.

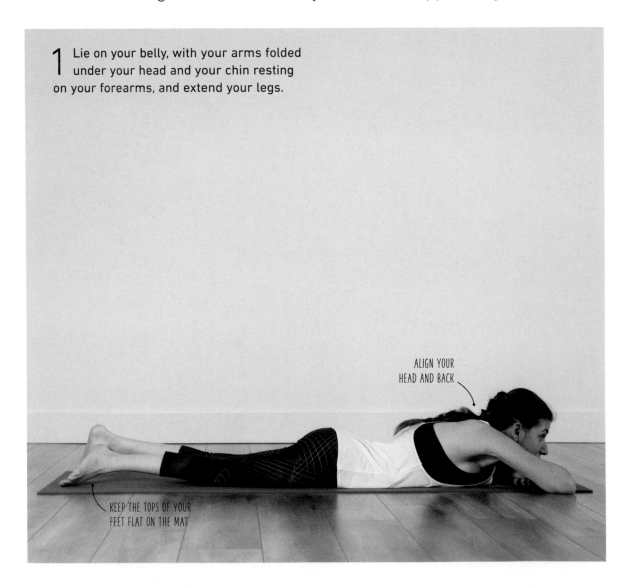

ALIGN YOUR HEAD AND BACK

KEEP THE TOPS OF YOUR FEET FLAT ON THE MAT

2 Place your hands at chest level and press down through your hands. Slightly lift your head off the mat, keeping your head and back aligned, and press your thighs together.

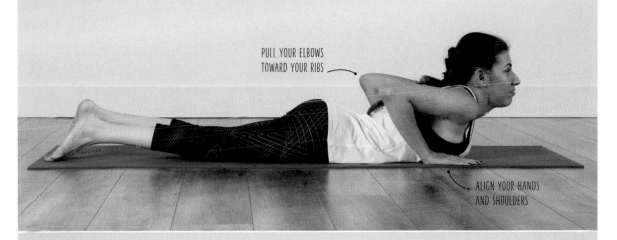

PULL YOUR ELBOWS TOWARD YOUR RIBS

ALIGN YOUR HANDS AND SHOULDERS

3 On an inhale, press your hands into the mat, curl your shoulders backward, and lift your upper body off the mat. Press your legs together, press down through the tops of your feet, and lift your chest forward. Hold this position for 3 to 5 full breaths.

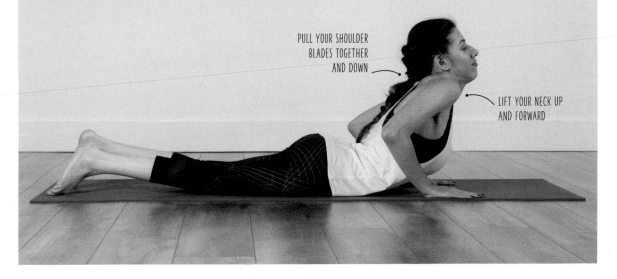

PULL YOUR SHOULDER BLADES TOGETHER AND DOWN

LIFT YOUR NECK UP AND FORWARD

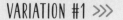

VARIATION #1 >>>

1. Stand facing a wall, with your arms straight and your hands flat on the wall.

2. Press through your hands, bend your elbows, lean your chest toward the wall, and curl your shoulders away from the wall. Hold this position for 3 to 5 full breaths.

ALIGN YOUR HANDS AND SHOULDERS

PULL YOUR UPPER BODY UP AND BACK

~COBRA~

VARIATIONS

People with sore or injured backs might find backbends challenging, making this pose inaccessible. But these variations can help you open muscles throughout your chest.

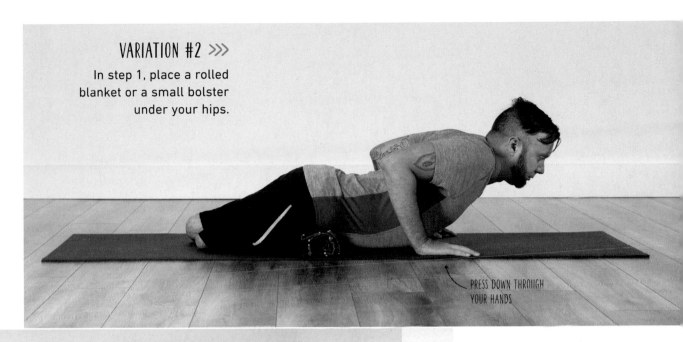

VARIATION #2 >>>

In step 1, place a rolled blanket or a small bolster under your hips.

PRESS DOWN THROUGH YOUR HANDS

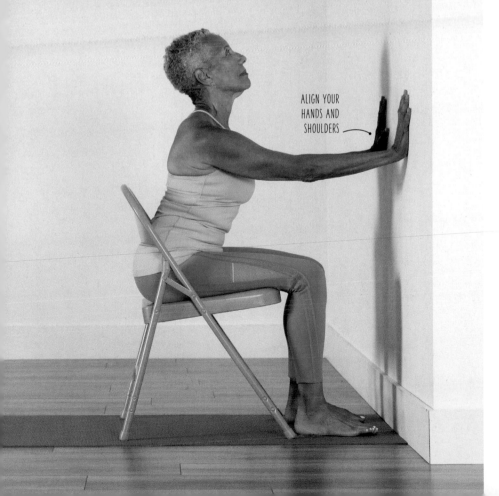

ALIGN YOUR HANDS AND SHOULDERS

<<< VARIATION #3

1. Sit in a chair facing a wall, with your feet flat on the mat and your arms relaxed at your sides.
2. Place your hands flat on the wall and lift your upper body up and back. Hold this position for 3 to 5 full breaths.

Bow

>>>DHANURASANA<<<

Fly like an arrow in this pose designed to strengthen your back muscles and stretch those muscles at the front of your body. These movements can also open the tight muscles of your quads and shoulders as well as stretch your abs.

1 Lie on your belly and extend your legs, with your head slightly lifted off the mat, the tops of your feet flat on the mat, and your arms relaxed at your sides.

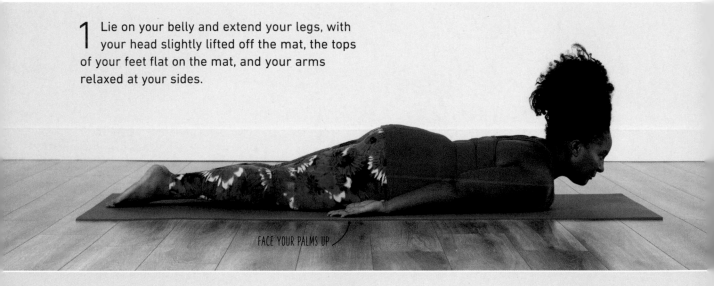

FACE YOUR PALMS UP

2 Bend your knees, reach your arms behind you, and grab your ankles with your hands. (Grab the outsides of your feet if that's easier.)

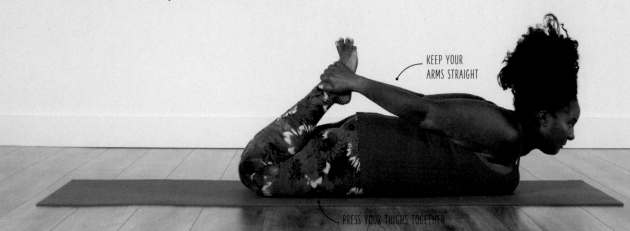

KEEP YOUR ARMS STRAIGHT

PRESS YOUR THIGHS TOGETHER

3 Press your ankles (or feet) into your hands and lift your thighs and chest off the mat, curling your shoulders backward and broadening across your collarbones. Press down through your pubic bone to pull yourself deeper into the backbend. Hold this position for 3 to 5 full breaths.

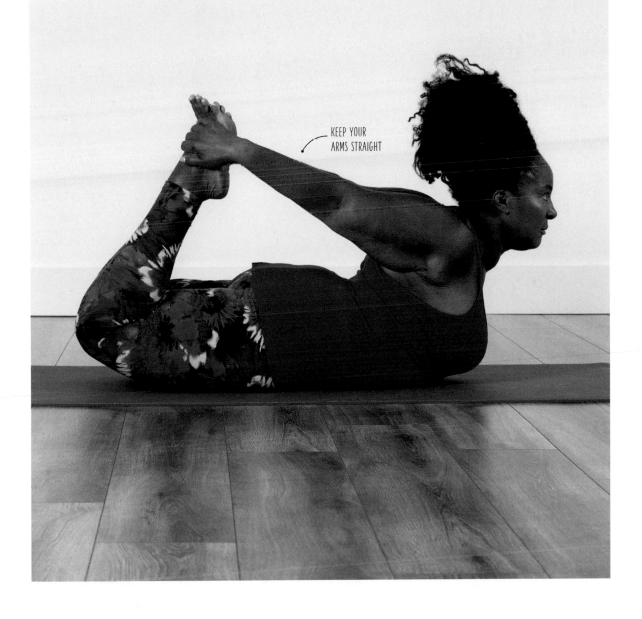

KEEP YOUR
ARMS STRAIGHT

~ B O W ~
VARIATIONS

If you have tight shoulders or lower-back discomfort,
try one of these alternative poses. Performing a variation
might even help ease some of that tension and allow you
to develop some strength in those areas.

≪≪ VARIATION #1

1. Lie on your right side, resting your left arm at your side
and resting your head on your right forearm and upper arm.
2. Bend your knees and bring your heel toward your buttocks.
Reach your left arm behind you and grab your left leg with
your left hand.
3. Push your left leg away from you and pull your left heel
toward your body. Hold this position for 3 to 5 full breaths.
Repeat these steps on the other side.

PUSH YOUR
ELBOWS INWARD

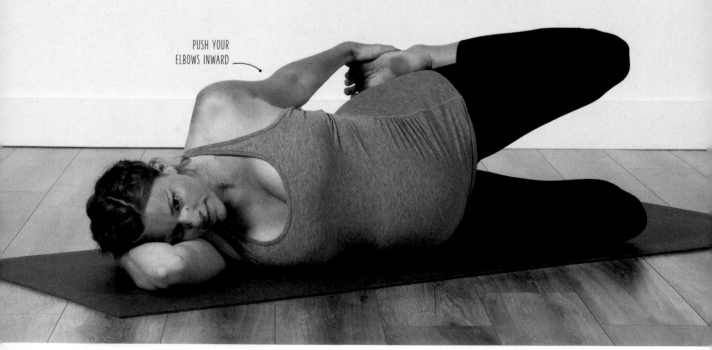

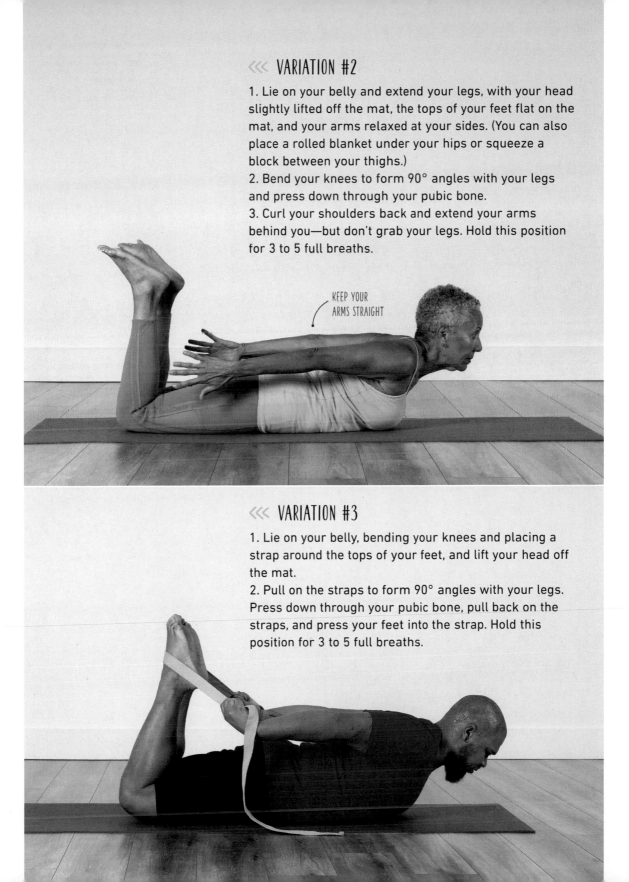

‹‹‹ VARIATION #2

1. Lie on your belly and extend your legs, with your head slightly lifted off the mat, the tops of your feet flat on the mat, and your arms relaxed at your sides. (You can also place a rolled blanket under your hips or squeeze a block between your thighs.)
2. Bend your knees to form 90° angles with your legs and press down through your pubic bone.
3. Curl your shoulders back and extend your arms behind you—but don't grab your legs. Hold this position for 3 to 5 full breaths.

KEEP YOUR
ARMS STRAIGHT

‹‹‹ VARIATION #3

1. Lie on your belly, bending your knees and placing a strap around the tops of your feet, and lift your head off the mat.
2. Pull on the straps to form 90° angles with your legs. Press down through your pubic bone, pull back on the straps, and press your feet into the strap. Hold this position for 3 to 5 full breaths.

Revolved Lunge

>>> PARIVRTTA ANJANEYASANA <<<

Engaging your spine and back muscles during this pose can improve your balance and posture. You can also engage your abdominal muscles, like your transverse and oblique abs, while your legs provide stability and endurance.

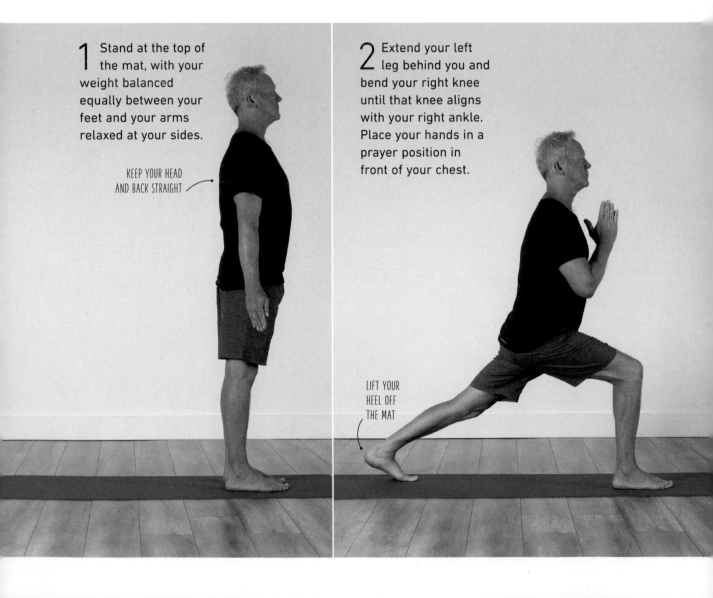

1 Stand at the top of the mat, with your weight balanced equally between your feet and your arms relaxed at your sides.

KEEP YOUR HEAD AND BACK STRAIGHT

2 Extend your left leg behind you and bend your right knee until that knee aligns with your right ankle. Place your hands in a prayer position in front of your chest.

LIFT YOUR HEEL OFF THE MAT

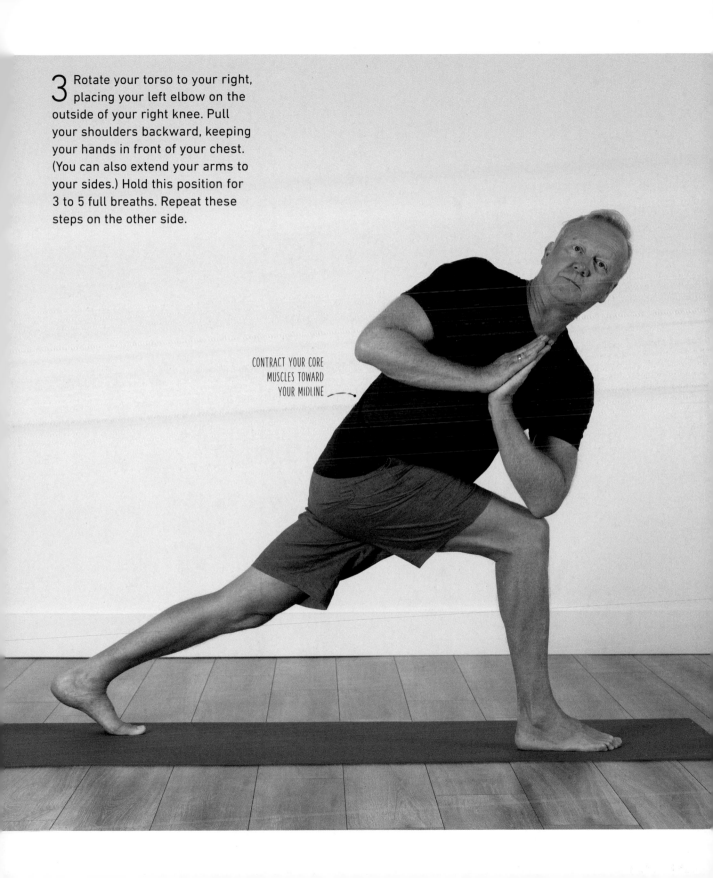

3 Rotate your torso to your right, placing your left elbow on the outside of your right knee. Pull your shoulders backward, keeping your hands in front of your chest. (You can also extend your arms to your sides.) Hold this position for 3 to 5 full breaths. Repeat these steps on the other side.

CONTRACT YOUR CORE MUSCLES TOWARD YOUR MIDLINE

~ REVOLVED LUNGE ~
VARIATIONS

Twisting your torso while maintaining the lunge in your lower body demands strength and balance. Using props, like a wall or blocks, can make this pose more accessible.

VARIATION #1 >>>

Place a block on its long edge near your left foot. In step 2, place your left hand on the block. In step 3, rotate your torso to your right, lifting your right arm toward the sky until aligned with your left arm. Hold this position for 3 to 5 full breaths. Repeat these steps on the other side.

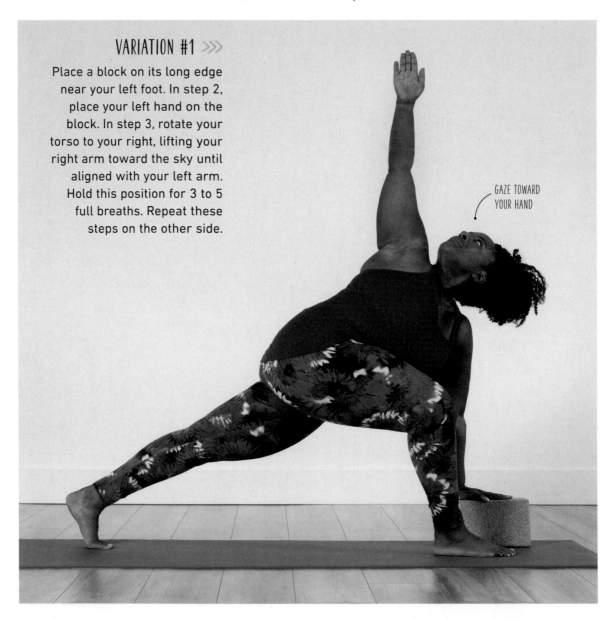

GAZE TOWARD YOUR HAND

VARIATION #2 »»»

In step 2, place your left knee on the mat. In step 3, rotate from beneath your rib cage, placing your left elbow on the outside of your right knee. (You can also place your left hand on a block.)

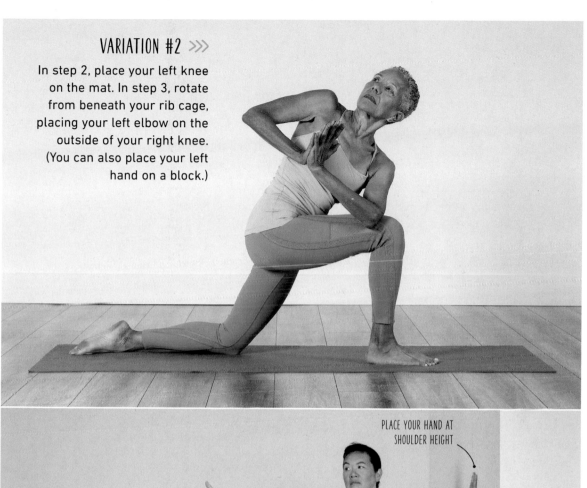

PLACE YOUR HAND AT SHOULDER HEIGHT

VARIATION #3 »»»

In step 1, stand facing a wall. In step 2, extend your left leg behind you and slightly bend your right knee. In step 3, rotate toward your right, place your left hand flat on the wall, and extend your right arm behind you until parallel with the mat.

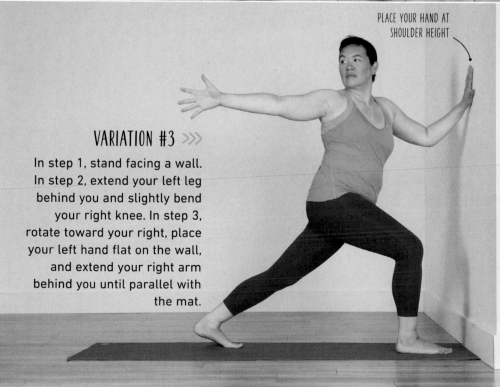

Cat-Cow

>>> MARJARIASANA–BITILASANA <<<

You can perform magic with this pose, transforming from
cow to cat using flowing movements that warm your body
and bring flexibility to your spine. This pose also invites
a connection between your breaths and your movements.

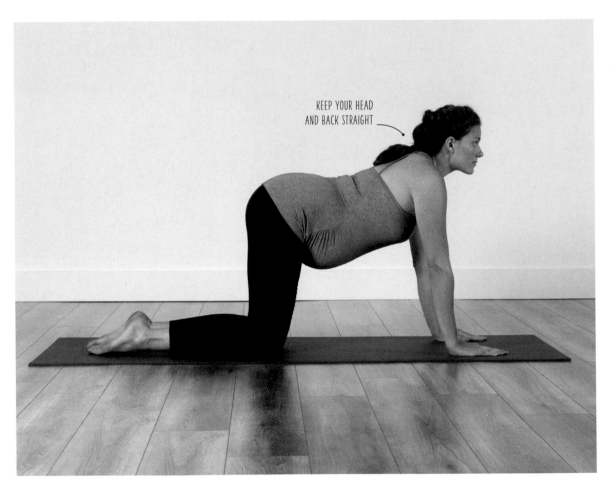

KEEP YOUR HEAD
AND BACK STRAIGHT

1 Place your hands, knees, and the tops of your feet flat on
the mat, with your hands slightly in front of your
shoulders, your knees slightly behind your hips, and your
index fingers pressed into the mat.

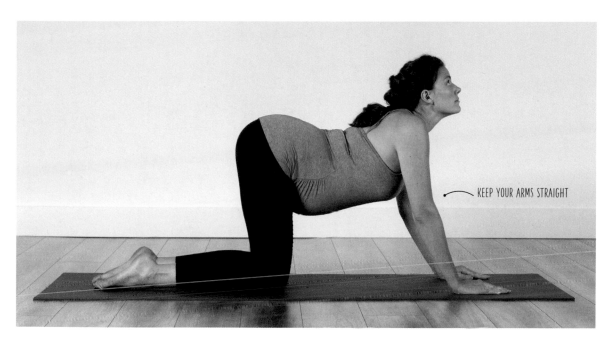

KEEP YOUR ARMS STRAIGHT

2 On an inhale, push your belly toward the mat, creating
a deep concave curve in your spine. Lift your sitting
bones toward the sky and broaden your collarbones forward.

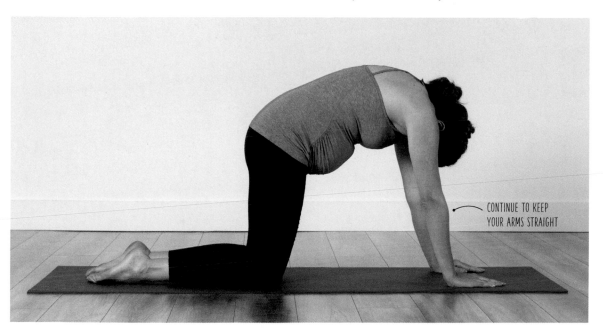

CONTINUE TO KEEP
YOUR ARMS STRAIGHT

3 On an exhale, press down through your hands and
strengthen your arms, pushing the mat away from you
and creating a strong convex curve. Hold this position for
3 to 5 full breaths.

~ CAT-COW ~
VARIATIONS

If you have physical challenges or limitations related to your back, these seated and standing variations might make this pose more accessible.

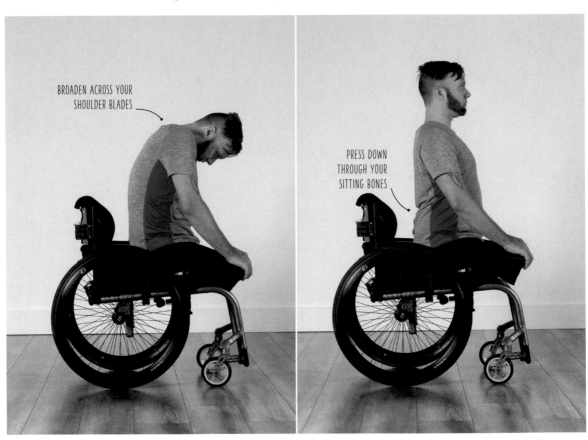

BROADEN ACROSS YOUR SHOULDER BLADES

PRESS DOWN THROUGH YOUR SITTING BONES

⋘ VARIATION #1

1. Sit on the edge of a chair, place your feet flat on the mat, and place your hands on your knees.
2. On an exhale, round your back and tuck your chin into your chest.
3. On an inhale, pull your shoulder blades together and down, lifting your chest forward. Hold this position for 3 to 5 full breaths.

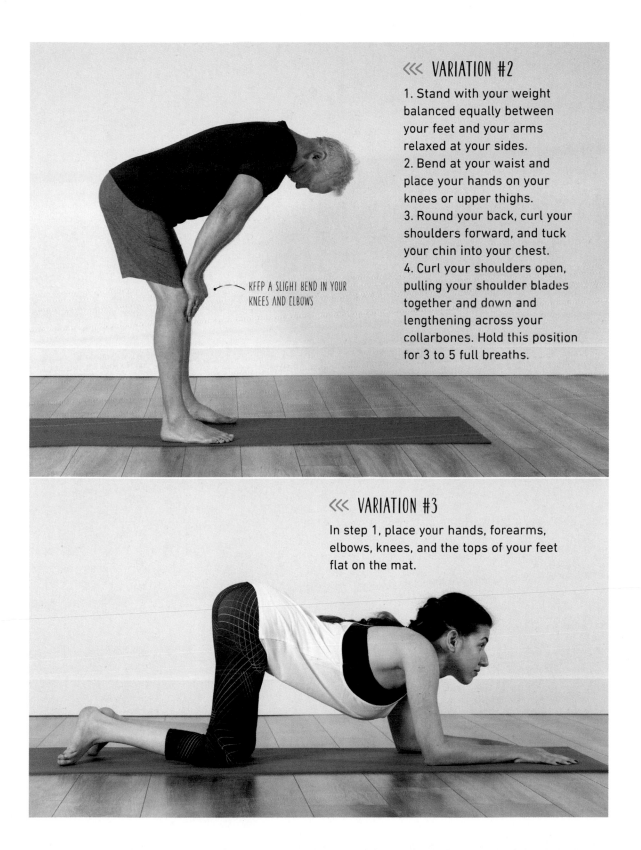

««« VARIATION #2

1. Stand with your weight balanced equally between your feet and your arms relaxed at your sides.
2. Bend at your waist and place your hands on your knees or upper thighs.
3. Round your back, curl your shoulders forward, and tuck your chin into your chest.
4. Curl your shoulders open, pulling your shoulder blades together and down and lengthening across your collarbones. Hold this position for 3 to 5 full breaths.

KEEP A SLIGHT BEND IN YOUR KNEES AND ELBOWS

««« VARIATION #3

In step 1, place your hands, forearms, elbows, knees, and the tops of your feet flat on the mat.

Sage

>>> PARIVRTTA MARICHYASANA <<<

This twist is a great way to lubricate the joints of your spine while also creating a sense of calm throughout your body. These movements massage several organs, which can increase blood flow when you release from this pose.

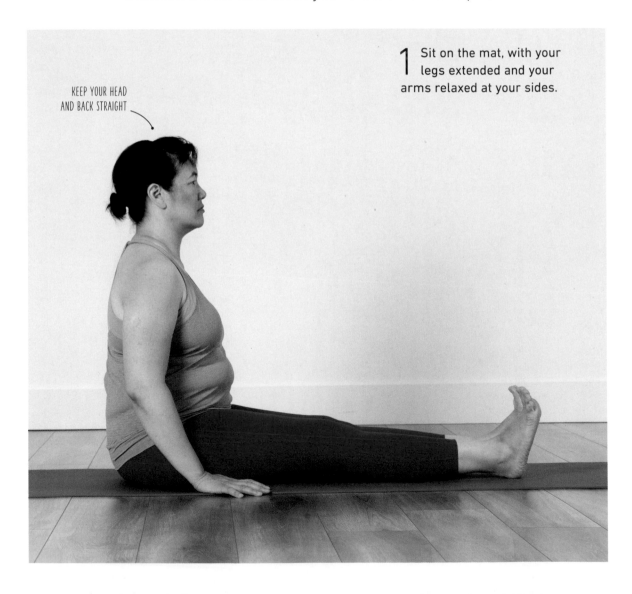

KEEP YOUR HEAD AND BACK STRAIGHT

1 Sit on the mat, with your legs extended and your arms relaxed at your sides.

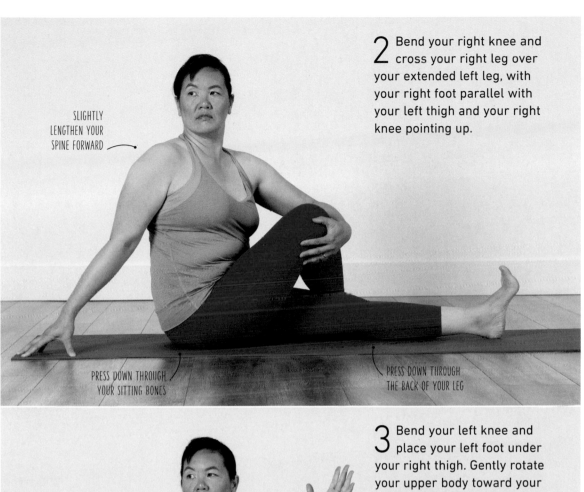

SLIGHTLY
LENGTHEN YOUR
SPINE FORWARD

2 Bend your right knee and cross your right leg over your extended left leg, with your right foot parallel with your left thigh and your right knee pointing up.

PRESS DOWN THROUGH
YOUR SITTING BONES

PRESS DOWN THROUGH
THE BACK OF YOUR LEG

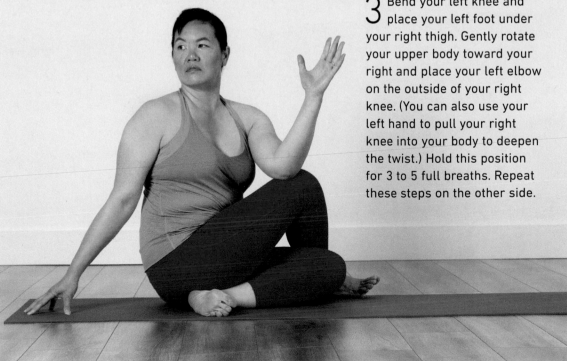

3 Bend your left knee and place your left foot under your right thigh. Gently rotate your upper body toward your right and place your left elbow on the outside of your right knee. (You can also use your left hand to pull your right knee into your body to deepen the twist.) Hold this position for 3 to 5 full breaths. Repeat these steps on the other side.

~ SAGE ~

VARIATIONS

Twists can prove challenging if you have an abundance
in the center of your body. Twists with a bind can also be
difficult if your arms aren't long enough to reach behind
you. These variations can help with these situations.

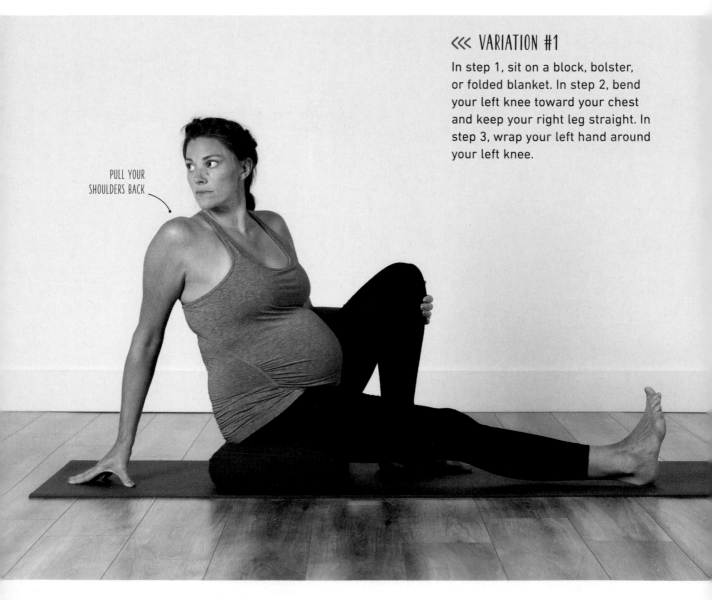

≪≪ VARIATION #1

In step 1, sit on a block, bolster,
or folded blanket. In step 2, bend
your left knee toward your chest
and keep your right leg straight. In
step 3, wrap your left hand around
your left knee.

PULL YOUR
SHOULDERS BACK

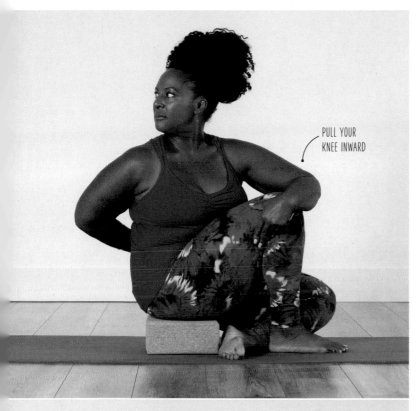

PULL YOUR
KNEE INWARD

‹‹‹ VARIATION #2

In step 1, sit on a block, bolster, or folded blanket. In step 2, tuck your left foot behind your right ankle and place your right arm behind your back. In step 3, place your left hand on the outside of your right knee.

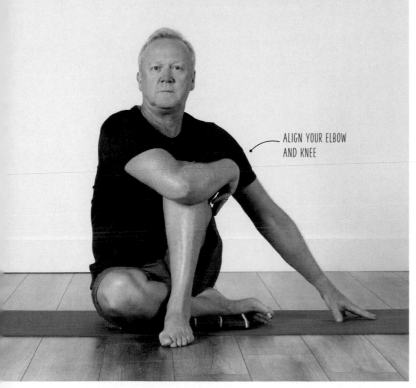

ALIGN YOUR ELBOW
AND KNEE

‹‹‹ VARIATION #3

1. Sit on the mat, with your legs extended and your arms relaxed at your sides. Place a folded blanket under your hips or sit on a bolster or a block.
2. Bend your left knee and bring your left leg to the inside of your right thigh. Bend your right knee and bring your right heel as close to your sitting bones as possible.
3. Bend your right elbow, reach around your left knee, and pull your left knee to your chest.
Hold this position for 3 to 5 full breaths. Repeat these steps on the other side.

GWEN

WHO IS GWEN JEUN?

I'm embracing my 51 years. I've been married for 21 years to the best guy ever. I was born in Ottawa and raised in Windsor, Ontario. I'm just a small animal veterinarian trying to live her yoga. I love food and cooking (especially baking bread), yoga and meditation, travel and a good book. And I'm addicted to my iPhone. I'm an advocate for wellness in the veterinary profession and I promote yoga as a tool for skillful living. I meet with a group of veterinary colleagues once a year to meditate and practice yoga. We stay in touch via an online weekly meditation group.

HOW DID YOU GET STARTED PRACTICING YOGA?

I took my first class with Dianne—when I was 39 years old! I don't consider myself an athlete, so I was happily surprised by what I was able to train my body to do with Dianne as my yoga teacher. I felt safe taking chances to explore my physical self in poses. I discovered meditation through classes at

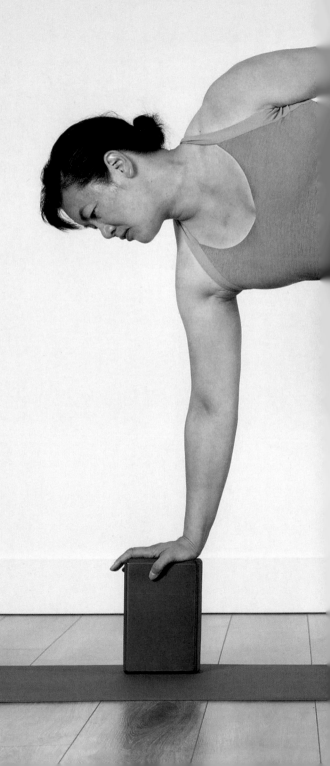

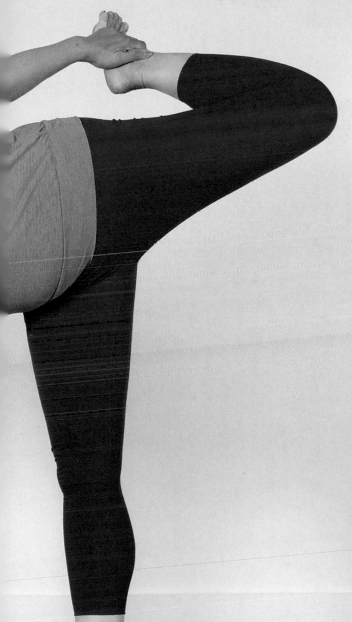

FAVORITE POSE
>>> HALF MOON

MOST CHALLENGING POSE
>>> TREE

OCCUPATION
>>> SMALL ANIMAL
VETERINARIAN

the studio and I've continued to study and read about it. I love practicing with Dianne—so much so that I took my yoga teacher training with her in 2011. I've enjoyed the opportunity to assist in her teacher training program, where I get to share my interest in yin yoga.

WHAT HAS PRACTICING YOGA TAUGHT YOU?

Yoga has taught me that having a daily meditation practice is good for my well-being. Developing a personal asana practice is challenging! My motivation is how good my body feels after I do a pose or two and it keeps me going. Breathing techniques (ujjayi, natural breath, square breathing) are also good to help me in stressful times. Paying attention to how my breath changes during a difficult pose reminds me to reassess what I'm doing and why and that it's only temporary. Learning to live inside my body—and not just inside the thoughts in my head—was the biggest lesson for me.

Revolved Fire Log

>>>PARIVRTTA AGNISTAMBHASANA<<<

This seated twisting pose stretches your spine, lower-back muscles, torso, shoulders, and chest. These movements can also help you feel—and enjoy!—powerful stretching in your knees, ankles, and hips.

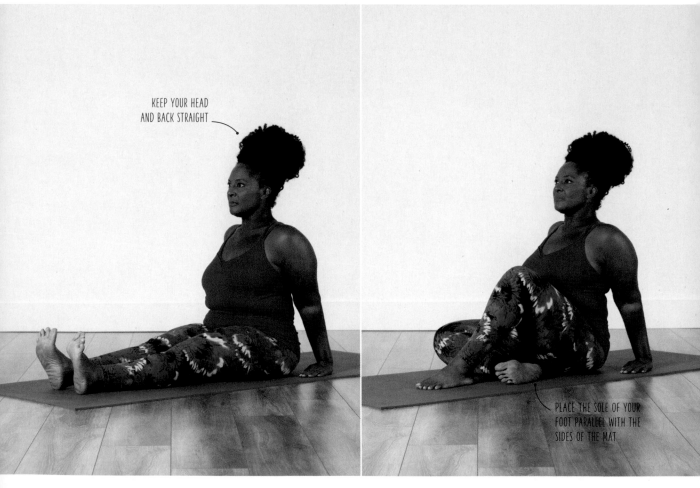

KEEP YOUR HEAD AND BACK STRAIGHT

PLACE THE SOLE OF YOUR FOOT PARALLEL WITH THE SIDES OF THE MAT

1 Sit in the middle of the mat, with your legs extended and your arms relaxed at your sides.

2 Bend your knees and slip your right leg under your left thigh until your right ankle and the back of your left ankle align.

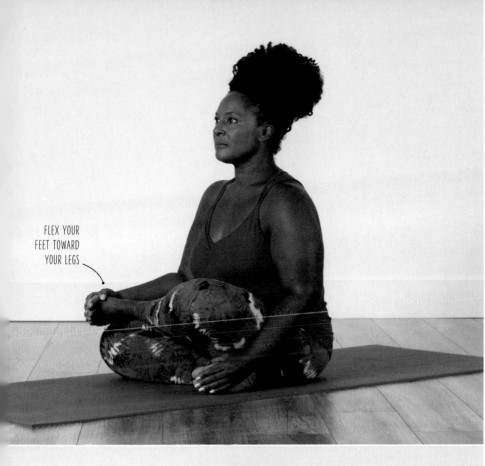

FLEX YOUR
FEET TOWARD
YOUR LEGS

3 Place your left
ankle on top of
your right knee,
keeping your upper
body parallel with the
top of the mat, and
place your hands on
the soles of your feet.

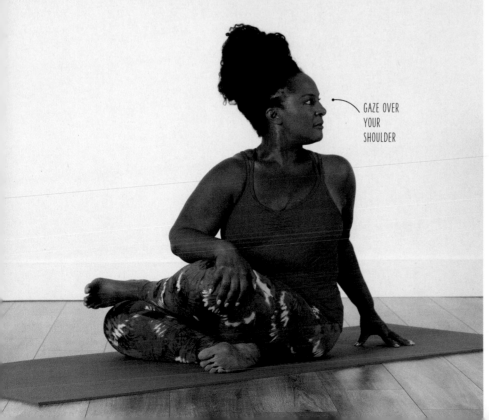

GAZE OVER
YOUR
SHOULDER

4 Place your left
hand on the mat
behind you and place
your right hand on the
outside of your left
knee. On an exhale,
gently rotate your
upper body to your
left. Hold this position
for 3 to 5 full breaths.
Repeat these steps on
the other side.

⌒ REVOLVED FIRE LOG ⌒
VARIATIONS

Because this is an advanced pose, it requires flexibility. Some knees can't handle the intense stretch these movements offer, but these variations can help you explore this pose without overexerting your knees and hip joints.

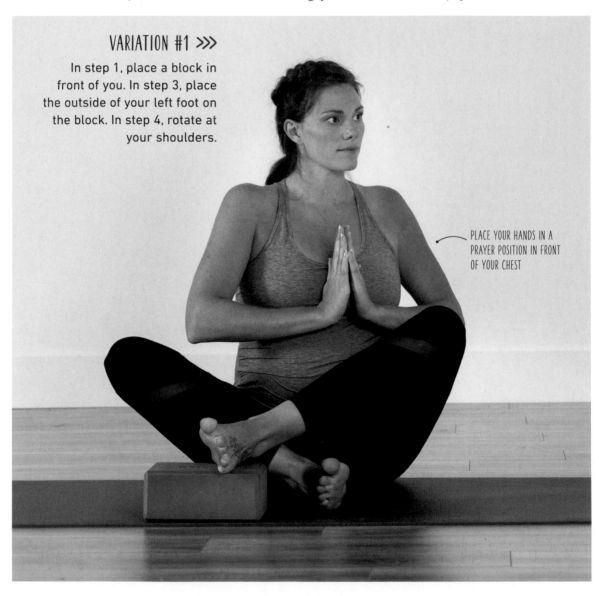

VARIATION #1 >>>

In step 1, place a block in front of you. In step 3, place the outside of your left foot on the block. In step 4, rotate at your shoulders.

PLACE YOUR HANDS IN A PRAYER POSITION IN FRONT OF YOUR CHEST

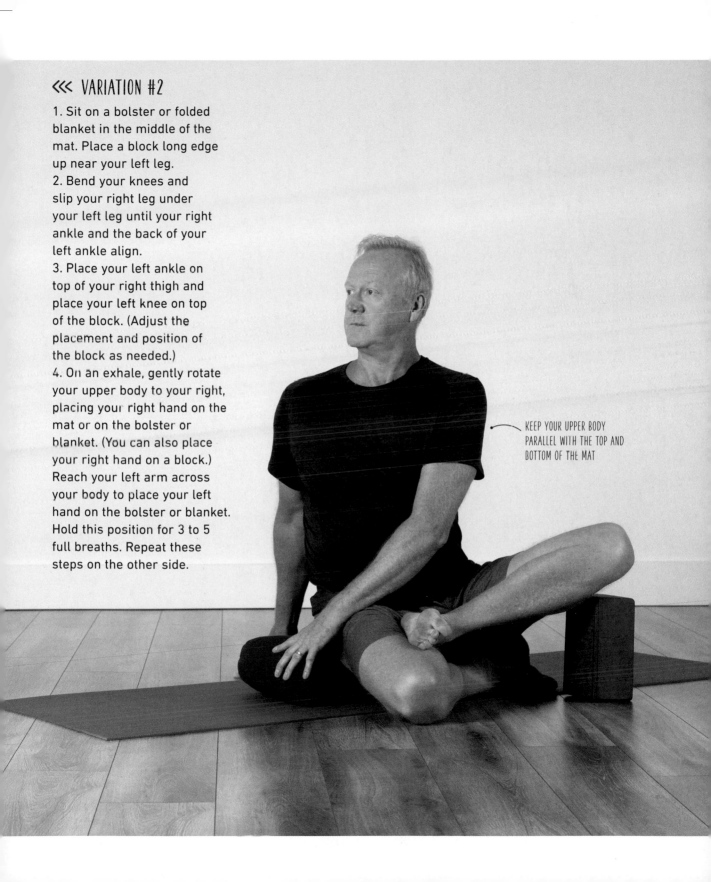

⫷⫷⫷ VARIATION #2

1. Sit on a bolster or folded blanket in the middle of the mat. Place a block long edge up near your left leg.

2. Bend your knees and slip your right leg under your left leg until your right ankle and the back of your left ankle align.

3. Place your left ankle on top of your right thigh and place your left knee on top of the block. (Adjust the placement and position of the block as needed.)

4. On an exhale, gently rotate your upper body to your right, placing your right hand on the mat or on the bolster or blanket. (You can also place your right hand on a block.) Reach your left arm across your body to place your left hand on the bolster or blanket. Hold this position for 3 to 5 full breaths. Repeat these steps on the other side.

KEEP YOUR UPPER BODY PARALLEL WITH THE TOP AND BOTTOM OF THE MAT

Revolved
Hand to Big Toe

>>> PARIVRTTA SUPTA PADANGUSTHASANA <<<

When you perform the movements in this pose, you can stretch muscles from your shoulders to your feet. This pose can also help improve your hamstring and spine flexibility, relieve pressure in your lower back, and aid with digestion.

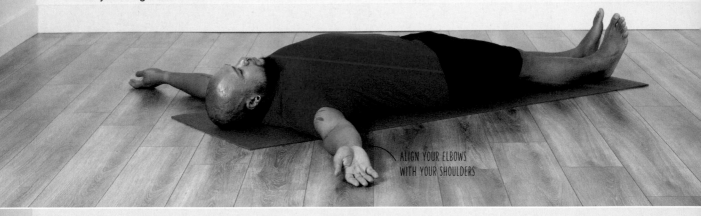

1 Lie on your back, with your arms extended to form a T and your legs extended.

ALIGN YOUR ELBOWS WITH YOUR SHOULDERS

2 Bend your left knee, bring your left leg toward your chest, and wrap your interlaced fingers below your left knee.

KEEP YOUR HEAD FLAT ON THE MAT

3 Grab your left big toe with your right index and middle fingers, slightly bend your left knee, and begin to pull your left leg across your body.

EXTEND YOUR LEFT
ARM TO YOUR LEFT

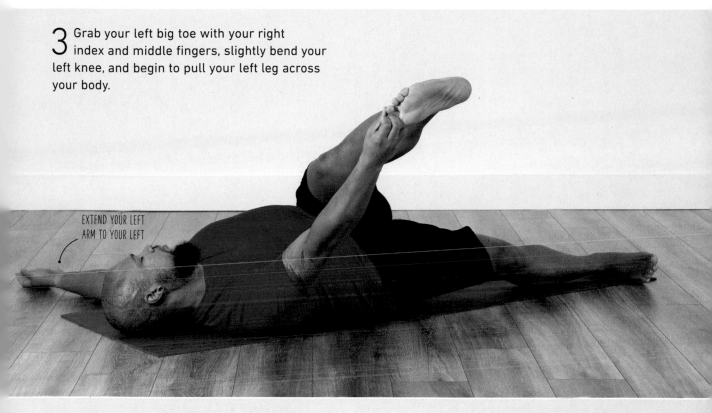

4 Continue to pull your left leg across your body until your foot is parallel with the sides of the mat. Hold this position for 3 to 5 full breaths. Repeat these steps on the other side.

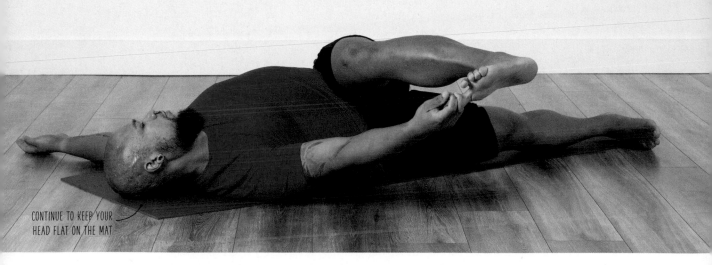

CONTINUE TO KEEP YOUR
HEAD FLAT ON THE MAT

∾ REVOLVED HAND TO BIG TOE ∾
VARIATIONS

Shorter arms and tight shoulder muscles can make these movements challenging. These variations can help this pose feel more accessible.

⋘ VARIATION #1

1. Lie on your back, with your knees bent, your legs pulled toward your chest, and your arms relaxed at your sides.

2. Extend your arms to form a T and extend your legs. (You can also bend your elbows to form a cactus shape.)

3. Rotate to your right and bring your left leg across your right leg until your left foot touches the floor and is parallel with the sides of the mat. (If your shoulders feel tight, you can also place your left hand on your left hip or place a folded blanket under your shoulders.) Hold this position for 3 to 5 full breaths. Repeat these steps on the other side.

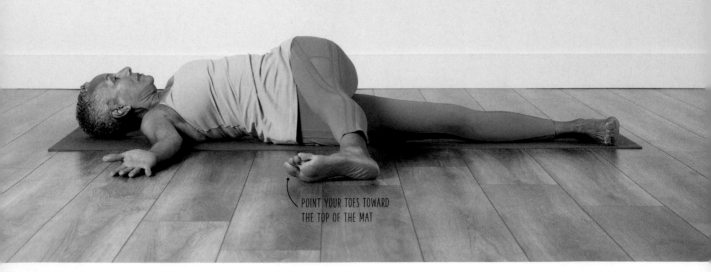

POINT YOUR TOES TOWARD
THE TOP OF THE MAT

≪≪ VARIATION #2

1. Lie on your back, with your arms extended to form a T and your legs extended.
2. Bend your left knee and bring your left leg toward your chest.
3. Place your right hand on your left knee and gently pull your left leg across your body toward your right. Keep your left hand at your waist or place a rolled blanket under your left shoulder. Hold this position for 3 to 5 full breaths. Repeat these steps on the other side.

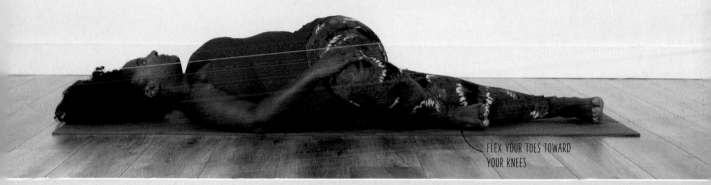

FLEX YOUR TOES TOWARD YOUR KNEES

≪≪ VARIATION #3

In step 1, loop a strap around the ball of your left foot. Use the strap in the remaining steps to pull and hold your left leg. (For added support, you can also place a block under your left foot.)

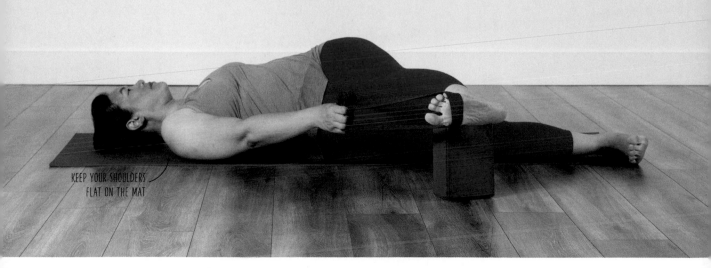

KEEP YOUR SHOULDERS FLAT ON THE MAT

Thread the Needle

>>> PARSVA BALASANA <<<

This take on Child's Pose offers a gentle twist that stretches and opens your shoulders, chest, arms, upper back, and neck. These movements can also relieve tightness in your upper back and between your shoulder blades.

1 Place your hands, knees, and the tops of your feet flat on the mat, with your wrists under or slightly in front of your shoulders and your knees under your hips.

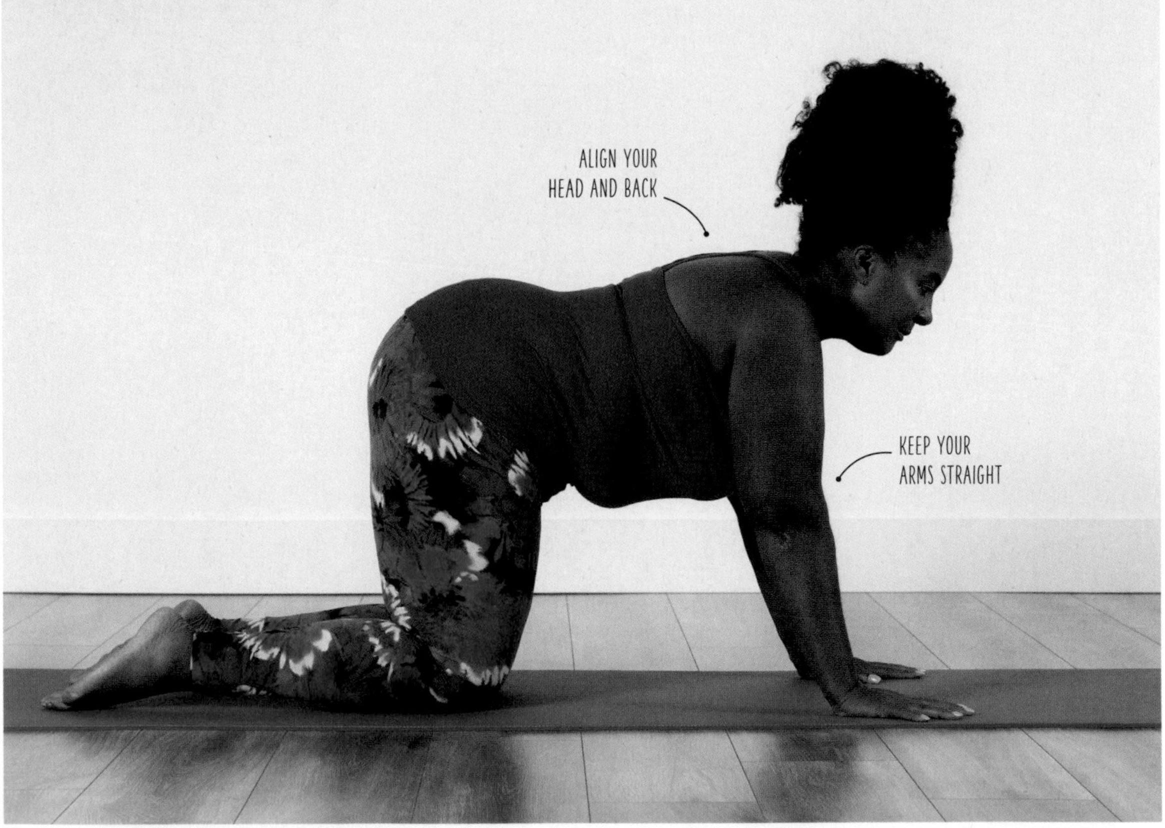

ALIGN YOUR
HEAD AND BACK

KEEP YOUR
ARMS STRAIGHT

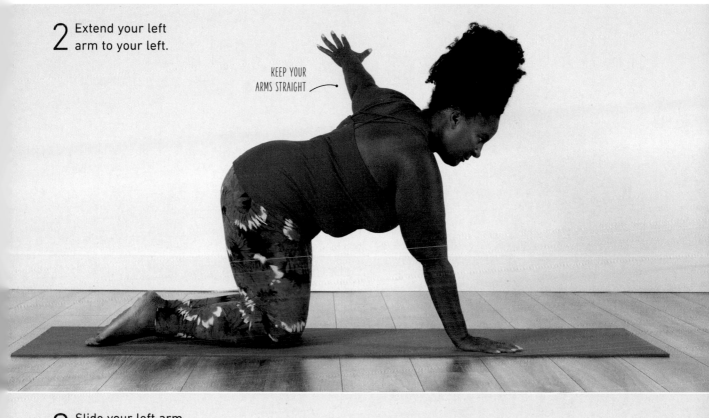

2 Extend your left arm to your left.

KEEP YOUR ARMS STRAIGHT

3 Slide your left arm under your chest and to your right. Place your left shoulder, ear, and cheek on the mat. Hold this position for 3 to 5 full breaths. Repeat these steps on the other side.

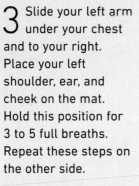

FACE YOUR PALM TOWARD THE SKY

∽ THREAD THE NEEDLE ∽
VARIATIONS

If you have tight or stiff muscles in your upper back
and shoulders, you might find this to be a difficult pose.
But using a block or a bolster can allow you to enjoy these
movements and gain similar benefits to the main pose.

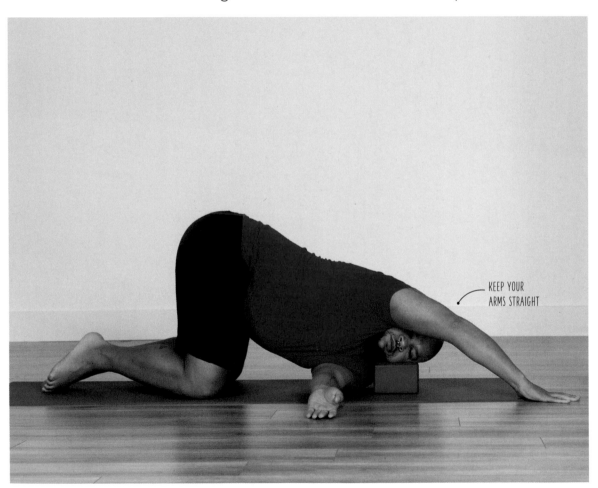

KEEP YOUR
ARMS STRAIGHT

⋘ VARIATION #1

In step 1, place a block long side up
below your head. In step 3, place
your head on the block and lower
yourself toward the mat.

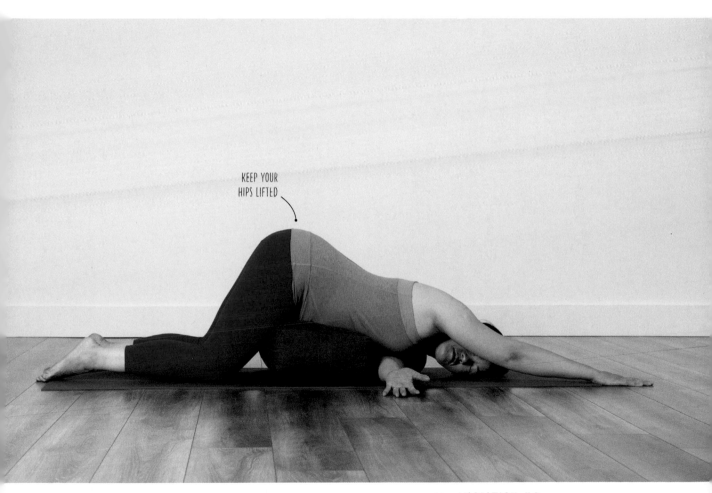

KEEP YOUR
HIPS LIFTED

‹‹‹ VARIATION #2

In step 1, place a bolster on the mat below your torso. In step 3, lower yourself onto the bolster.

Seated Forward Fold

>>> PASCHIMOTTANASANA <<<

If you need relaxing movements that stretch your lower back, glutes, and hamstrings, this pose is for you. Forward folds naturally pull your focus inward, helping soothe your central nervous system and calm your mind.

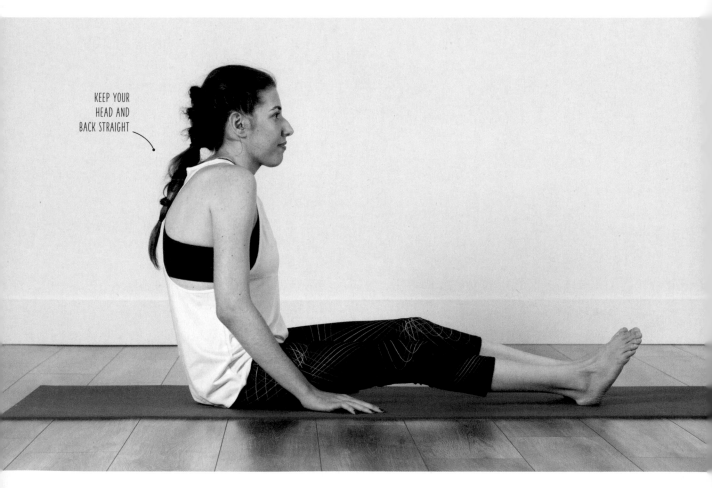

KEEP YOUR HEAD AND BACK STRAIGHT

1 Sit on the mat, with your legs extended, a slight bend in your knees, and your arms relaxed at your sides. (You can also sit on a folded blanket.)

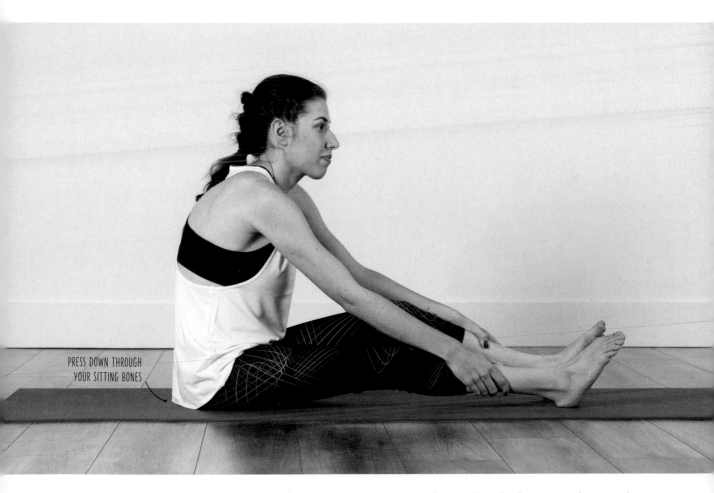

PRESS DOWN THROUGH
YOUR SITTING BONES

2 Bend at your waist, walk your hands down your legs, and
lean your chest toward your knees. Stop folding when
you first feel a stretch in your lower back, glutes, or
hamstrings. Hold this position for 3 to 5 full breaths.

∽ SEATED FORWARD FOLD ∽
VARIATIONS

Making some slight adjustments to the movements
of this pose can help extend how deeply you fold.
And you can still reap similar benefits to the main pose.

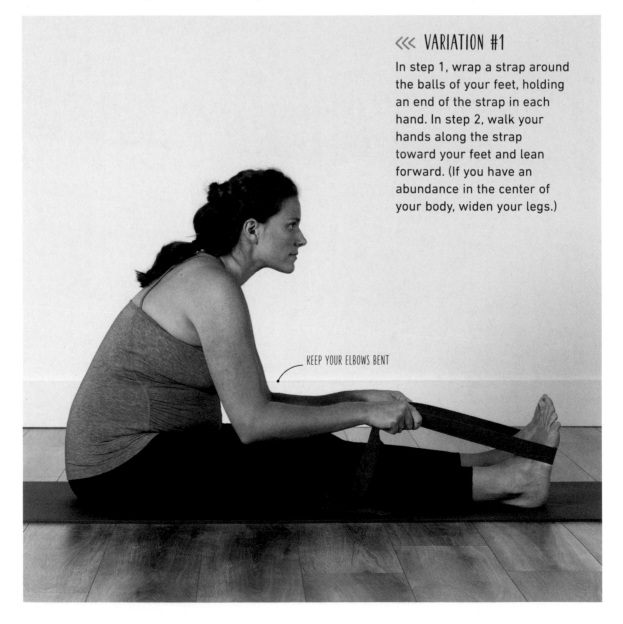

⫷ VARIATION #1

In step 1, wrap a strap around
the balls of your feet, holding
an end of the strap in each
hand. In step 2, walk your
hands along the strap
toward your feet and lean
forward. (If you have an
abundance in the center of
your body, widen your legs.)

KEEP YOUR ELBOWS BENT

⫷⫷⫷ VARIATION #2

1. Sit cross-legged on the mat, with your hands resting on your thighs. Place a block short edge up on the mat in front of you.
2. Bend at your waist and extend your arms, walking your hands forward until you place your head on the block. Hold this position for 3 to 5 full breaths.

ALLOW YOUR BACK
TO CURVE SLIGHTLY

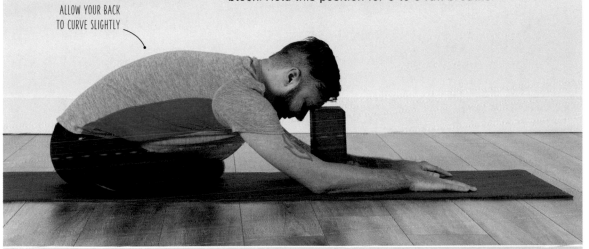

⫷⫷⫷ VARIATION #3

In step 1, place a rolled blanket under your knees. In step 2, walk your hands toward your feet, wrap your hands around your feet, and lean forward.

REST YOUR ELBOWS
ON THE BLANKET

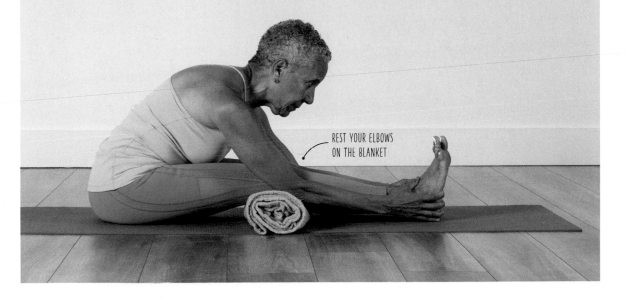

Locust

>>> SALABHASANA <<<

Focused on strengthening your deep core and back muscles, this backbending pose can also help lengthen and extend your spine. When done properly, this pose can provide therapeutic benefits for your lower back.

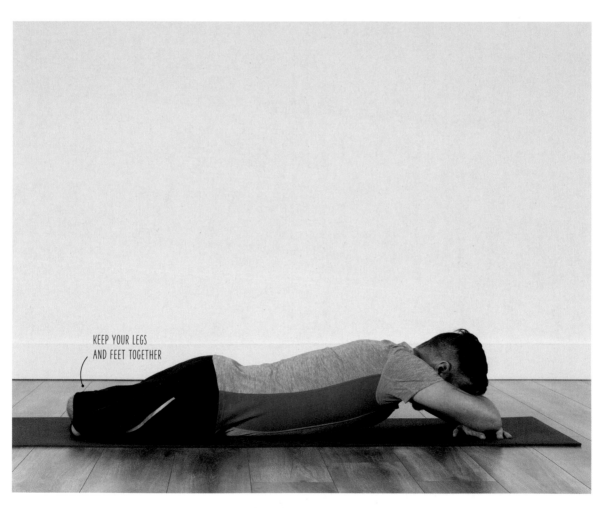

KEEP YOUR LEGS AND FEET TOGETHER

1 Lie on your belly, with your legs extended, your arms stacked under your head, and your head resting on your forearms.

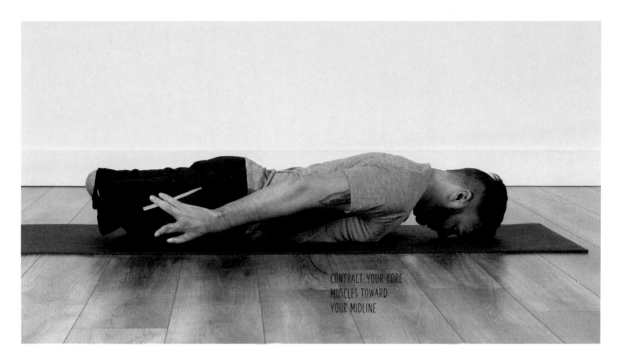

CONTRACT YOUR CORE
MUSCLES TOWARD
YOUR MIDLINE

2 On an inhale, extend your arms down
your sides and lift your lower legs off the
mat, keeping your upper legs flat on the mat.

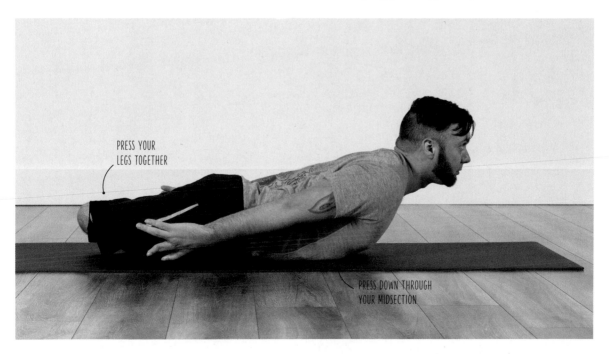

PRESS YOUR
LEGS TOGETHER

PRESS DOWN THROUGH
YOUR MIDSECTION

3 Lift your chest off the mat. Hold this position
for 3 to 5 full breaths.

∽LOCUST∽
VARIATIONS

Building strength in your back and core can help
reduce back pain. This pose is a great way to help keep
your spine healthy and more flexible, and these variations
can help you achieve those goals.

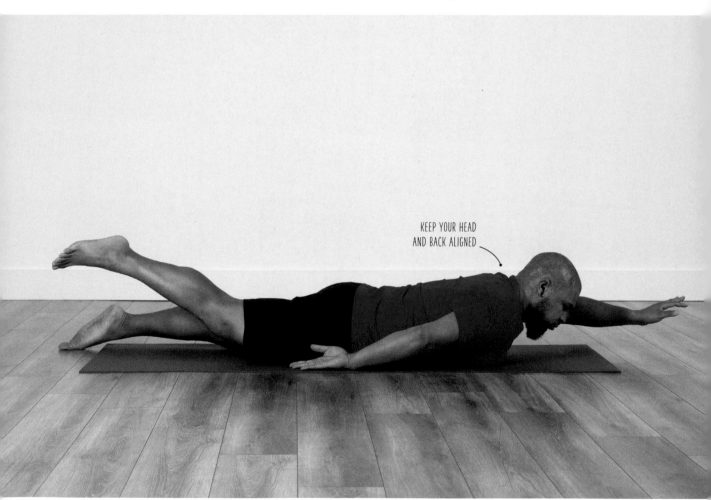

KEEP YOUR HEAD
AND BACK ALIGNED

⟨⟨⟨ VARIATION #1

In steps 2 and 3, alternate lifting opposite arms
and legs. For example, lift your left arm and lift
your right leg.

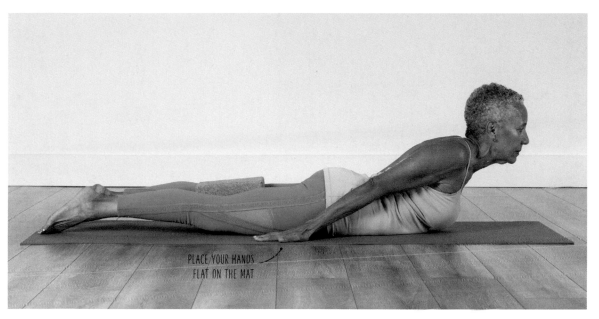

PLACE YOUR HANDS
FLAT ON THE MAT

‹‹‹ VARIATION #2

In step 1, place a block between your upper thighs. In step 2, squeeze the block and lift only your upper body off the mat.

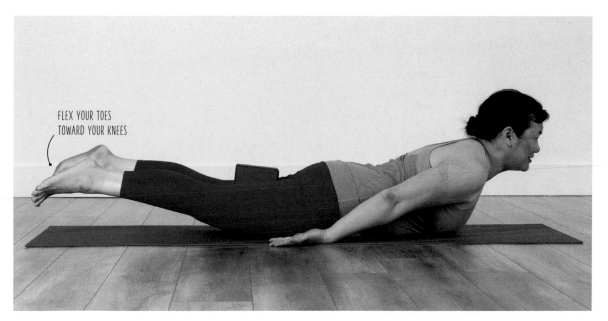

FLEX YOUR TOES
TOWARD YOUR KNEES

‹‹‹ VARIATION #3

In step 1, place a block between your upper thighs. In step 2, squeeze the block and focus on lifting your legs off the mat.

Shoulder Stand

>>> SARVANGASANA <<<

This inversion pose stretches your neck and shoulders while strengthening your abdominal and leg muscles. Performing these movements might also offer therapeutic properties to your thyroid gland and respiratory system.

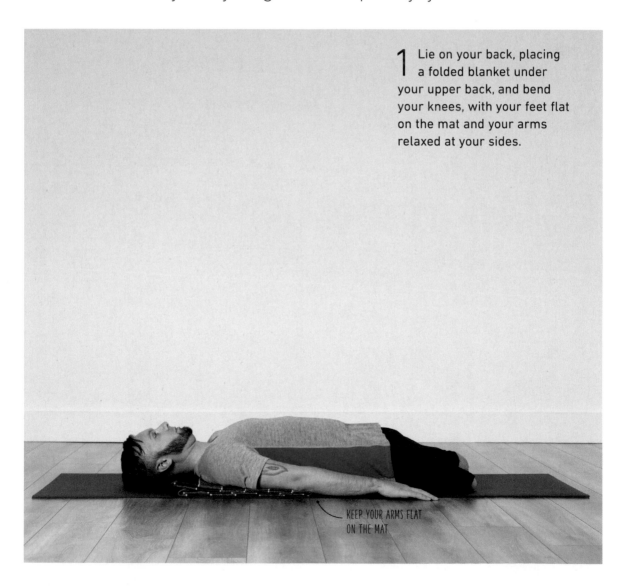

1 Lie on your back, placing a folded blanket under your upper back, and bend your knees, with your feet flat on the mat and your arms relaxed at your sides.

KEEP YOUR ARMS FLAT ON THE MAT

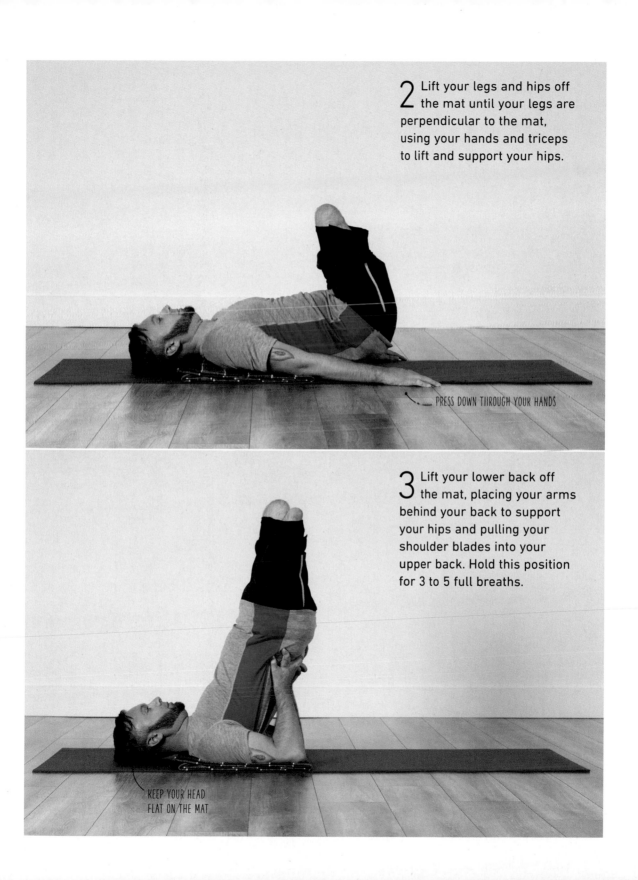

2 Lift your legs and hips off the mat until your legs are perpendicular to the mat, using your hands and triceps to lift and support your hips.

PRESS DOWN THROUGH YOUR HANDS

3 Lift your lower back off the mat, placing your arms behind your back to support your hips and pulling your shoulder blades into your upper back. Hold this position for 3 to 5 full breaths.

KEEP YOUR HEAD FLAT ON THE MAT

∼ SHOULDER STAND ∼
VARIATIONS

Finding balance in this pose is especially challenging for individuals with neck or shoulder injuries. Try these accessible variations to enjoy some of the therapeutic benefits of this pose without compromising your neck or shoulder muscles.

⫷ VARIATION #1

1. Place a chair in the middle of the mat, with the seat facing toward the back of the mat, and place a folded blanket on the mat. Sit sideways in the chair and rotate your body to slide your legs over the back of the chair.

2. Keeping your legs on the back of the chair, reach your hands behind you and grab the chair legs. Slide backward toward the back of the mat and rest your shoulders on the folded blanket. Allow the seat of the chair to support your lower back. Hold this position for 3 to 5 full breaths.

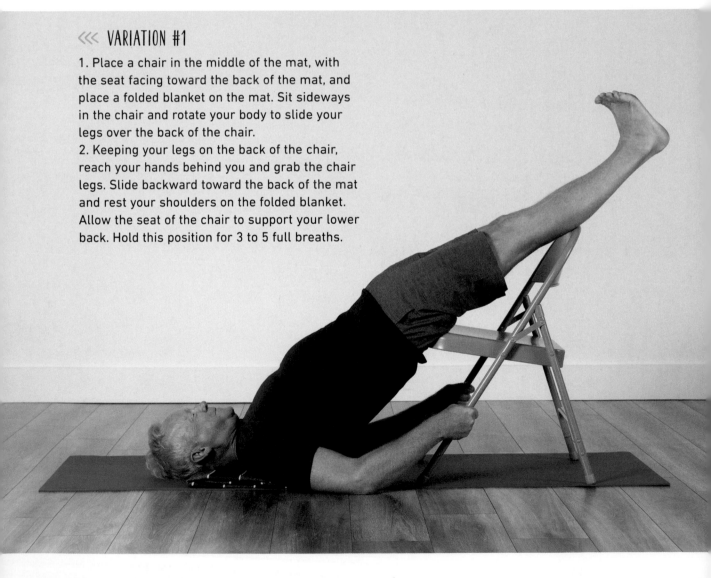

VARIATION #2 >>>

In step 1, place the short end of the mat near a wall, place a block nearby, and place the soles of your feet against a wall. In step 2, bend your knees, lift your hips, and place the block under your hips. In step 3, bring the backs of your thighs parallel with the wall.

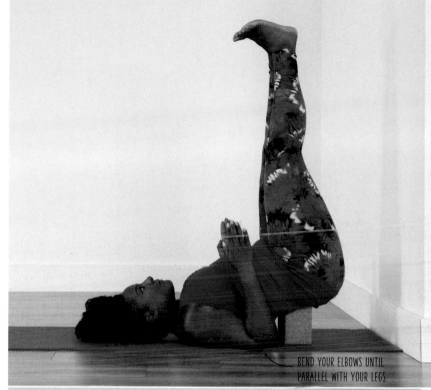

BEND YOUR ELBOWS UNTIL PARALLEL WITH YOUR LEGS

VARIATION #3 >>>

In step 1, place the short end of the mat near a wall and place a folded blanket in the middle of the mat. Use the blanket to support your upper back as you perform the remaining steps, continuing to keep your feet flat on the wall.

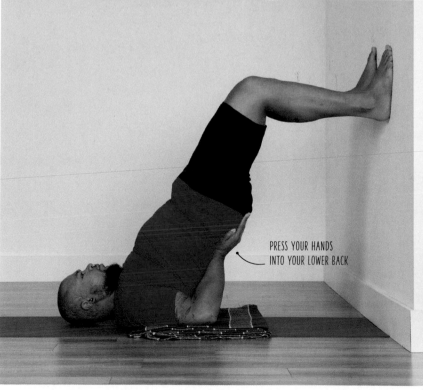

PRESS YOUR HANDS INTO YOUR LOWER BACK

JOHN

WHO IS JOHN AZLEN?

I work as an optical clerk. This is a job I truly enjoy because I work in a fun, fast-paced environment with a great group of coworkers who make it feel more like family than work. I enjoy the challenge of finding the right kind of frame to suit each customer.

I'm also a public speaker. In my presentations, I talk about overcoming real and personal barriers, accessibility, and ways to easily increase access for everyone. I also talk about the importance of living an active lifestyle.

I'm a community activist, peer mentor, and an accessibility advocate. I'm the co-founder of a peer support program for amputees and their families in my community. In this position, I use my personal experiences to help new amputees understand that they can still live the life they want—it just might look a little different than they imagined. They might need to learn to do things in a different way, but amputation doesn't have to be a barrier to achieving their goals.

After encountering a lack of options in my community, I also co-founded a para-sports club, Rose City Riot, with the goal of increasing accessible opportunities for sports and recreation.

I'm passionate about my participation in these

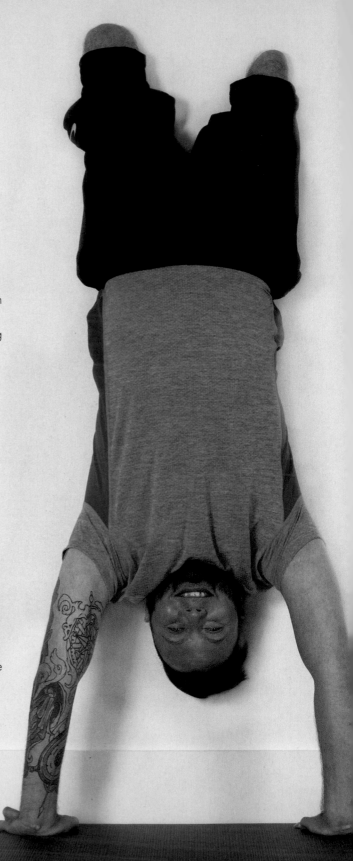

organizations and strive to actively engage my surrounding community. I raise awareness about the services and supports available to individuals with disabilities as well as the need for increased accessibility awareness.

In my spare time, I like to travel with my fiancé, go kayaking, take photographs, play wheelchair basketball, listen to live music, and play the occasional video game.

HOW DID YOU GET STARTED PRACTICING YOGA?

Preparing for this book was the first time I've done yoga. It was intimidating at first because I really didn't know what I was doing. As I began to feel more comfortable with the various poses, I started to enjoy it more. What I enjoyed most about this was that feeling of accomplishment—that one we all experience when we set the bar high and realize we can do anything as long as we put in the effort to reach our goals.

Yoga has been a discussion topic among the members of my amputee group and we've been looking for a local instructor to work with us. So when the opportunity to participate in *Yoga for Everyone* came up, I viewed this as a great chance to get started and learn yoga.

WHAT OBSTACLES HAVE YOU FACED IN YOGA AND HOW HAVE YOU RESPONDED TO THEM?

As I'm just beginning practicing yoga, I'm finding the aspect of balance to be my greatest challenge. Because I'm an amputee, my body is disproportionately top heavy, which I'm finding difficult to adjust to in certain poses (Boat pose specifically). As I continue on this journey, I know that my hyper-focus on my balance and posture will benefit me not only in yoga but also in my daily life in terms of strength and mobility.

I would also like to say that success feels so much better than fear. Never stop trying to succeed.

FAVORITE POSE
>>> SUPPORTED HANDSTAND

MOST CHALLENGING POSE
>>> BOAT

OCCUPATION
>>> OPTICAL CLERK

Bridge

>>> SETU BANDHA SARVANGASANA <<<

This pose is great for stretching your chest, neck, spine, and hips. These movements are also excellent for alleviating back pain, strengthening your buttock and hamstring muscles, and aiding with digestion.

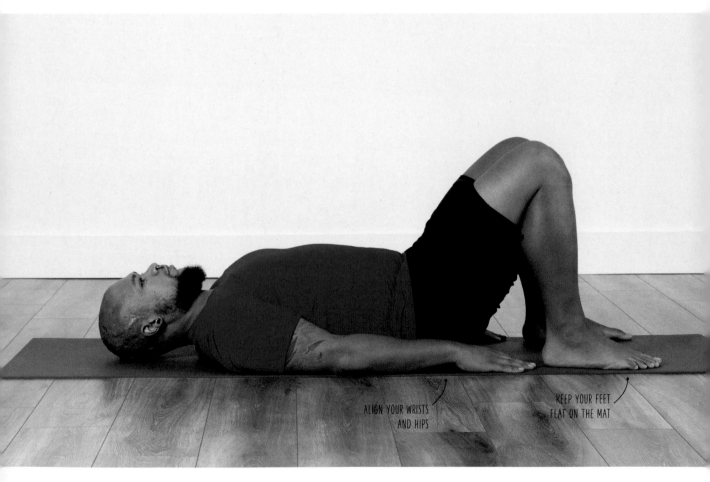

ALIGN YOUR WRISTS
AND HIPS

KEEP YOUR FEET
FLAT ON THE MAT

1 Lie on your back, with your knees bent, your heels as close to your body as possible, and your arms relaxed at your sides.

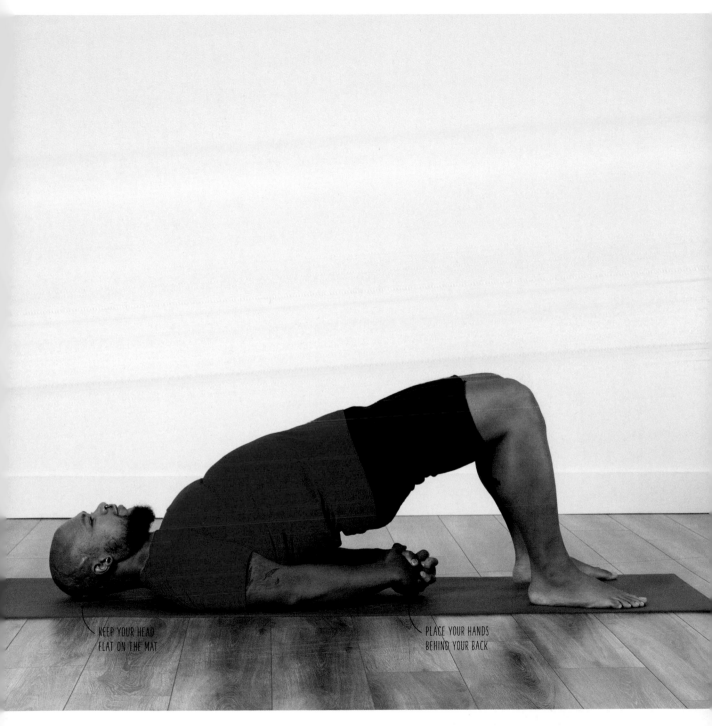

KEEP YOUR HEAD
FLAT ON THE MAT

PLACE YOUR HANDS
BEHIND YOUR BACK

2 Press down through your feet and use your leg muscles, glutes, and pelvic floor to lift your hips toward the sky. Hold this position for 3 to 5 full breaths.

～ BRIDGE ～
VARIATIONS

Several variations can help make this pose more accessible. You can use a wall, the mat, and even a strap to help you safely explore—and enjoy!—this pose.

⫷ VARIATION #1

In step 2, grab the edges of the mat with your hands to help lift your hips a little higher. Pull the mat like you're trying to stretch it wide.

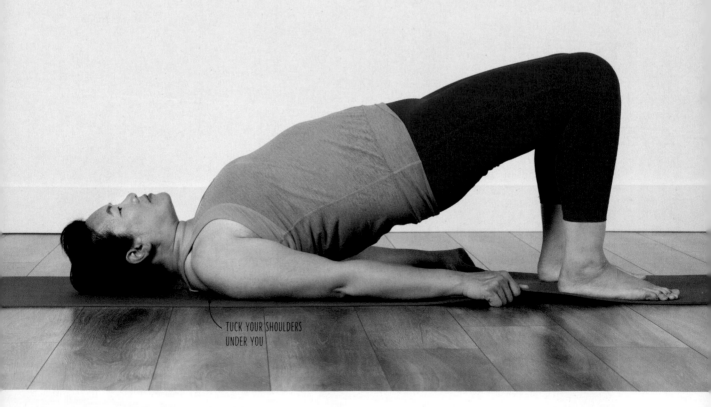

TUCK YOUR SHOULDERS
UNDER YOU

VARIATION #2 >>>

In step 2, place a block or two long edges up under your hips. (Adjust the placement and position of the blocks as needed. You can also place a block between your thighs to help engage your quads. In step 2, squeeze the block between your thighs and lift your hips.)

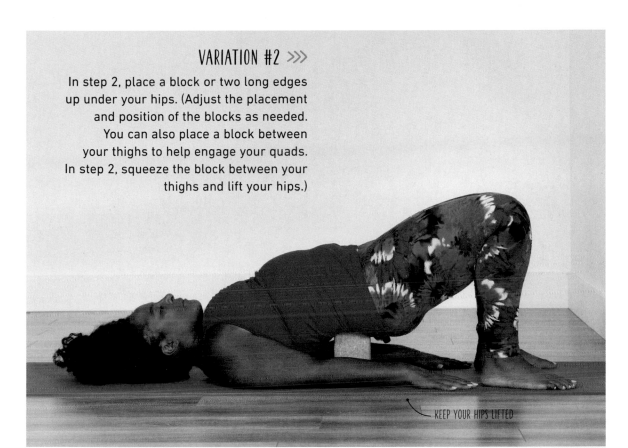

KEEP YOUR HIPS LIFTED

VARIATION #3 >>>

In step 1, place your knees flat against a wall or a chair.

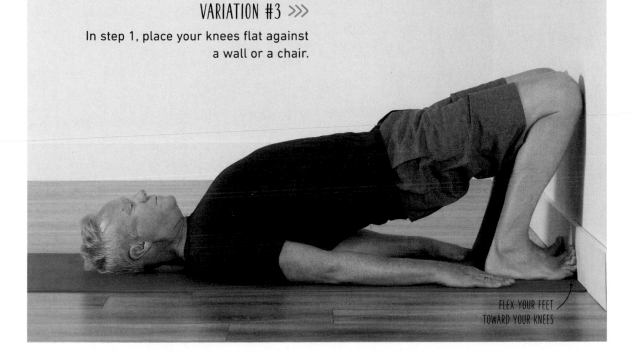

FLEX YOUR FEET
TOWARD YOUR KNEES

Supported Headstand

>>>SALAMBA SIRSASANA<<<

This pose can feel a little or a lot intimidating. Standing on your head can be terrifying and exhilarating, but because this pose can also strengthen your whole body and soothe your central nervous system, enjoy the experience.

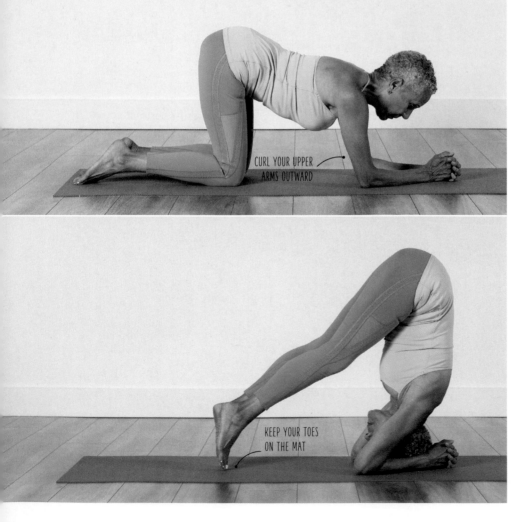

CURL YOUR UPPER ARMS OUTWARD

KEEP YOUR TOES ON THE MAT

1 Place your elbows, forearms, and knees flat on the mat and lace your fingers together, with your wrists pressed into the mat.

2 Place the crown of your head on the mat and place the back of your head against your intertwined fingers. Lift your knees off the mat and walk your feet toward your torso to form an inverted V with your body.

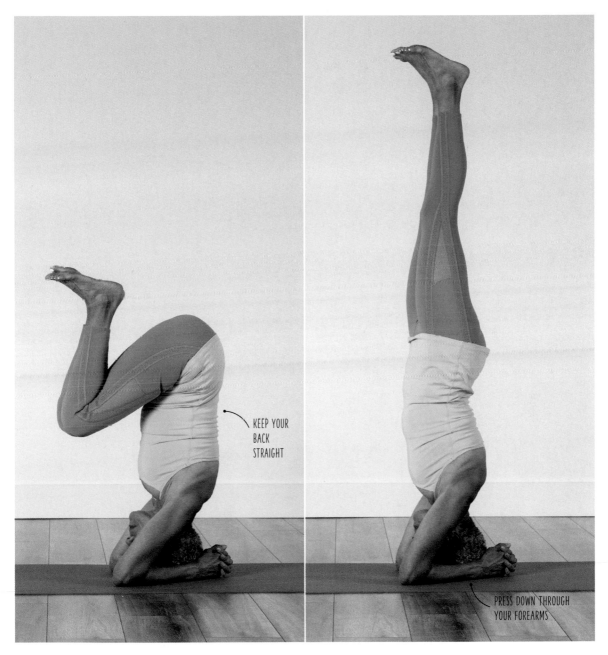

KEEP YOUR
BACK
STRAIGHT

PRESS DOWN THROUGH
YOUR FOREARMS

3 Press down through your forearms, walk your feet toward your body, and bend your knees and lift them toward your chest. Maintain your balance by pressing through your forearms and squeezing your belly. (You might need to perform these two actions a few times until you can maintain your balance with your knees bent and pulled toward your chest.)

4 Once you feel balanced, simultaneously and slowly extend your legs toward the sky. Take your time and move slowly. Hold this position for 3 to 5 full breaths.

∽ SUPPORTED HEADSTAND ∽
VARIATIONS

Headstands require exceptional strength in your
upper-body and core muscles. They're especially difficult
for people who can't place any weight on their heads
or cervical spine. But using a prop can help you safely
practice this pose while still protecting your neck and spine.

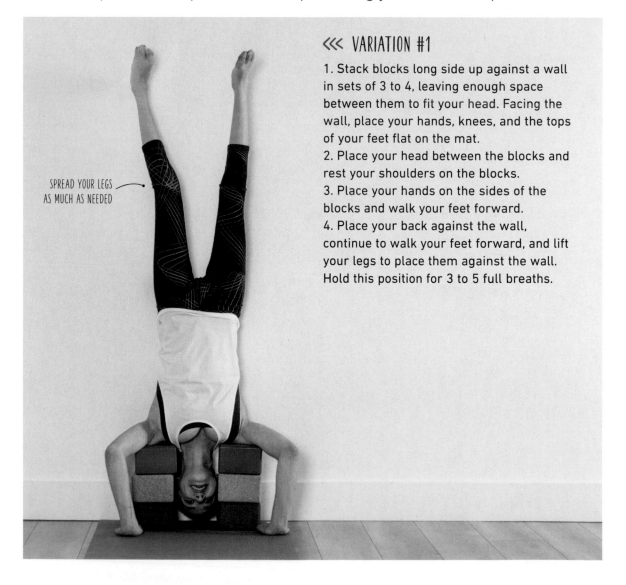

SPREAD YOUR LEGS
AS MUCH AS NEEDED

⟨⟨⟨ VARIATION #1

1. Stack blocks long side up against a wall
in sets of 3 to 4, leaving enough space
between them to fit your head. Facing the
wall, place your hands, knees, and the tops
of your feet flat on the mat.
2. Place your head between the blocks and
rest your shoulders on the blocks.
3. Place your hands on the sides of the
blocks and walk your feet forward.
4. Place your back against the wall,
continue to walk your feet forward, and lift
your legs to place them against the wall.
Hold this position for 3 to 5 full breaths.

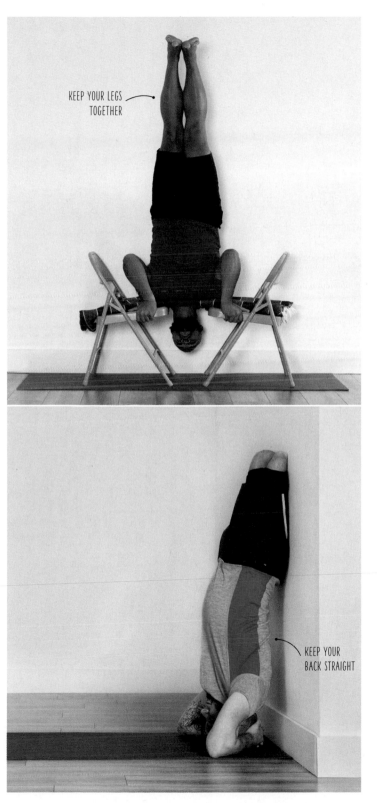

KEEP YOUR LEGS TOGETHER

KEEP YOUR BACK STRAIGHT

⫷ VARIATION #2

1. Place the longest edge of the mat against a wall. Place two chairs against the wall, with the seats facing each other, leaving enough space between the chairs for your head. Place a folded blanket on each seat.
2. Facing the wall, place your hands, knees, and the tops of your feet flat on the floor in front of the mat.
3. Place your head between the seats, rest your shoulders on the blankets, and grab the outer edges of the chairs with your hands.
4. Lift your legs toward the wall and place your back flat against the wall. Hold this position for 3 to 5 full breaths.

⫷ VARIATION #3

1. Facing a wall, place your hands, knees, and the tops of your feet flat on the mat. Intertwine your fingers and rest the back of your head in your hands.
2. Walk your feet toward the wall, place your back against the wall, and lift your legs toward your chest. Use the wall to maintain your balance and extend your legs toward the sky. Hold this position for 3 to 5 full breaths.

Sphinx

>>> SALAMBA BHUJANGASANA <<<

This pose might not help you walk like an Egyptian, but it can help open your chest, lungs, and lower back. Because you'll use your forearms for support, this pose is great if you have wrist pain, wrist injuries, or carpal tunnel syndrome.

1 Lie on your belly, with your arms stacked, your forearms and the tops of your toes flat on the mat, and your legs extended.

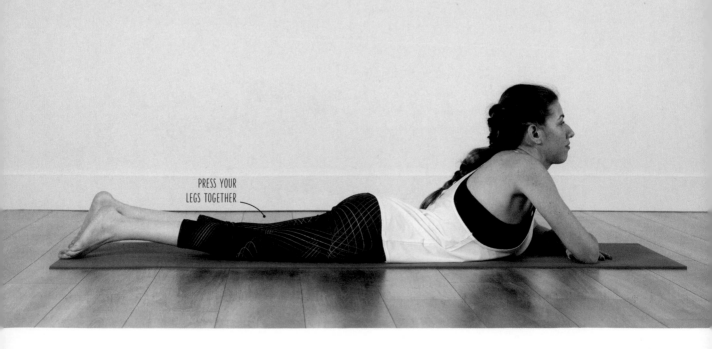

PRESS YOUR LEGS TOGETHER

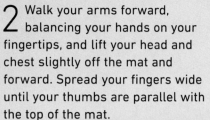

2 Walk your arms forward, balancing your hands on your fingertips, and lift your head and chest slightly off the mat and forward. Spread your fingers wide until your thumbs are parallel with the top of the mat.

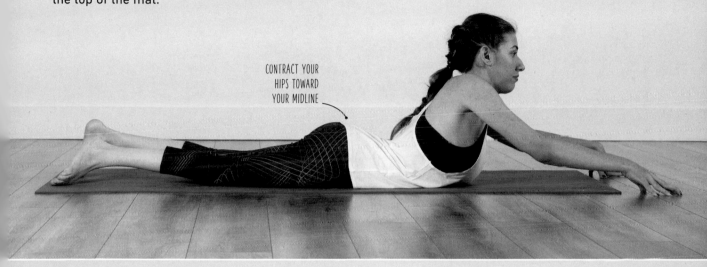

CONTRACT YOUR HIPS TOWARD YOUR MIDLINE

3 Place your forearms flat on the mat, press down through your forearms, and arch your back a little more. Pull your shoulder blades together and down, and broaden across your collarbones. Lengthen your tailbone toward your heels and press your pubic bone into the mat. Hold this position for 3 to 5 full breaths.

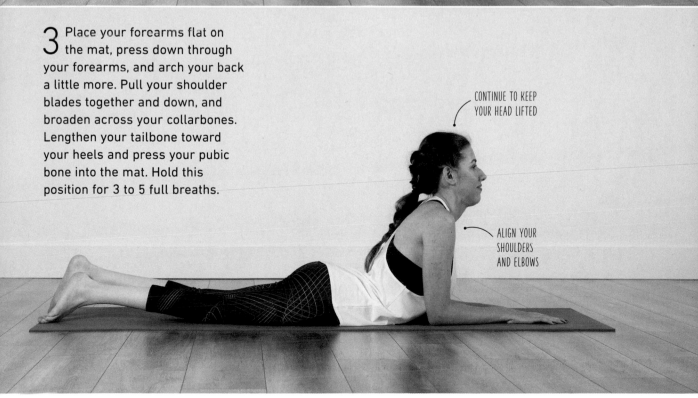

CONTINUE TO KEEP YOUR HEAD LIFTED

ALIGN YOUR SHOULDERS AND ELBOWS

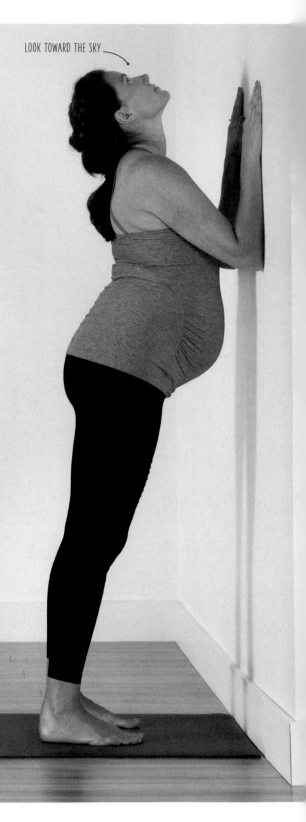

LOOK TOWARD THE SKY

~SPHINX~
VARIATIONS

Bending your back in any way can feel painful if you have an injured or sensitive lower back. These variations can help build strength and relieve some pressure in your lower back.

VARIATION #1 >>>

1. Stand facing a wall, with your forearms and hands flat against the wall, keeping your torso and feet from touching the wall.
2. Press your forearms against the wall and pull your shoulder blades together and down. Hold this position for 3 to 5 full breaths.

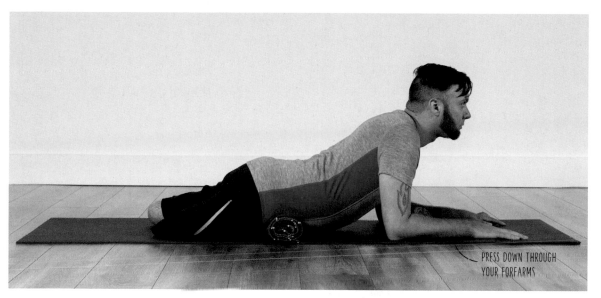

PRESS DOWN THROUGH YOUR FOREARMS

⋘ VARIATION #2

In step 1, place a small bolster or a rolled blanket under your hips.

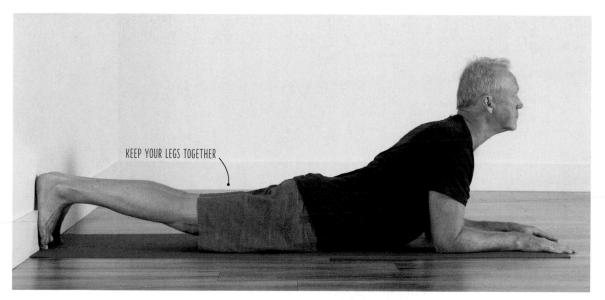

KEEP YOUR LEGS TOGETHER

⋘ VARIATION #3

1. Face away from a wall and lie on your belly, with your head and forearms flat on the mat and your feet flat against the wall.
2. Press down through your hips and forearms to lift your upper body off the mat. Hold this position for 3 to 5 full breaths.

Wheel

>>>URDHVA DHANURASANA<<<

When you're ready for the ultimate advanced backbend,
try this pose. These movements can open up your chest,
abdominal muscles, groin, and quads while also
strengthening your glutes, hamstrings, calves, and arms.

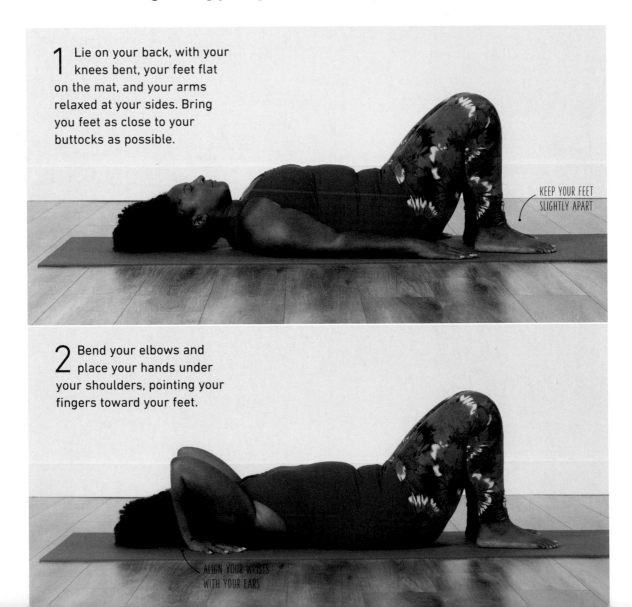

1 Lie on your back, with your knees bent, your feet flat on the mat, and your arms relaxed at your sides. Bring you feet as close to your buttocks as possible.

KEEP YOUR FEET SLIGHTLY APART

2 Bend your elbows and place your hands under your shoulders, pointing your fingers toward your feet.

ALIGN YOUR WRISTS WITH YOUR EARS

3 Press down through your hands and feet, lift your hips off the mat, and keep your head flat on the mat. (Reposition your hands wider if necessary.)

KEEP YOUR ELBOWS
SLIGHTLY BENT

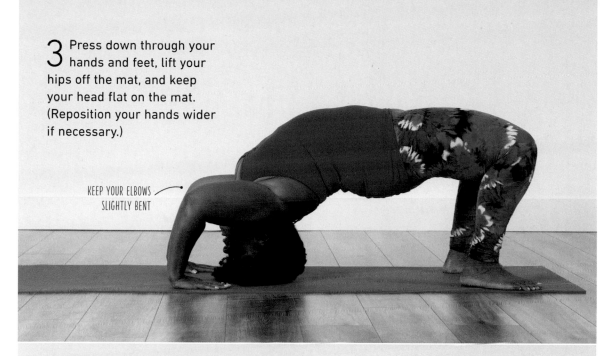

4 Press down through your legs and arms, lifting your head off the mat. Lift your chest up and back, straightening your arms and legs as much as possible. Hold this position for 3 to 5 full breaths.

ALIGN
YOUR FEET
AND KNEES

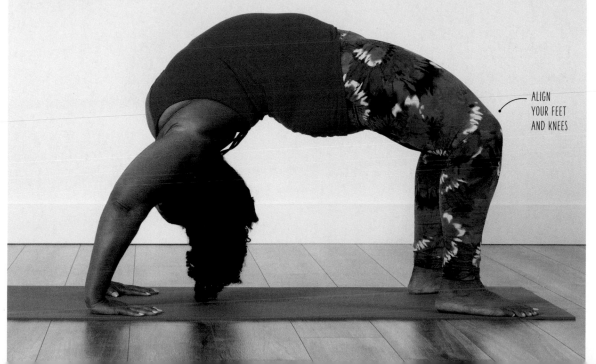

~WHEEL~
VARIATIONS

This pose can put pressure on your shoulders and wrists.
Because you need a lot of upper-body strength to perform
these movements, using props, like a ball, a blanket,
or a wall, can help create more accessible variations.

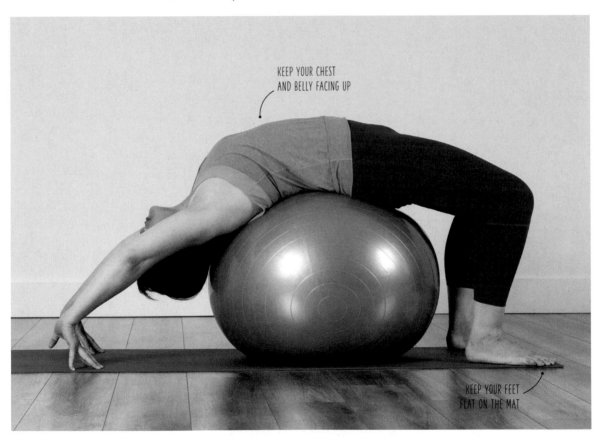

KEEP YOUR CHEST
AND BELLY FACING UP

KEEP YOUR FEET
FLAT ON THE MAT

⫷ VARIATION #1

1. Place an exercise ball on the mat and sit comfortably on
the ball to maintain your balance.
2. Place your hands on your waist, lean back and walk your
feet forward, and support your back on the ball.
3. Once you feel supported, extend your arms overhead and
behind you, lowering yourself until you touch the mat with
your fingertips. Hold this position for 3 to 5 full breaths.

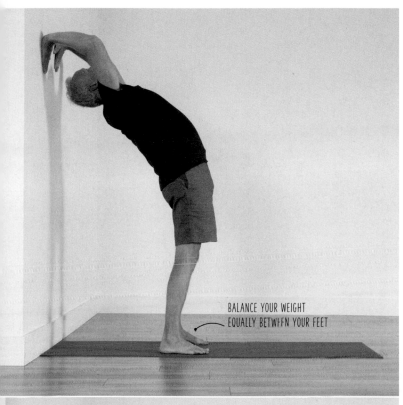

BALANCE YOUR WEIGHT
EQUALLY BETWEEN YOUR FEET

≪≪ VARIATION #2

1. Stand with your back against a wall. Place your hands on your hips and press down through your feet. Pull your legs apart energetically and pull your shoulder blades together and down.

2. Extend your arms overhead and behind you, placing your hands flat on the wall behind you.

3. Walk your hands down the wall and walk your feet away from the wall. Stop when you've stretched as far as comfortable. Hold this position for 3 to 5 full breaths.

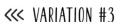

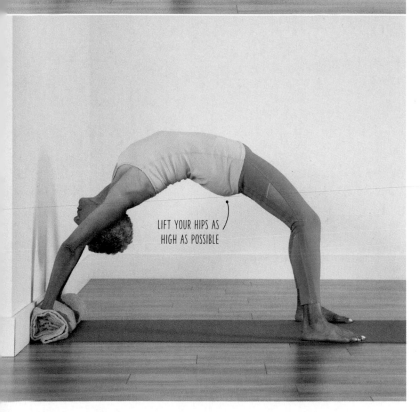

LIFT YOUR HIPS AS
HIGH AS POSSIBLE

≪≪ VARIATION #3

1. Place a rolled blanket or a small bolster against the base of a wall. Facing away from the wall, lie on your back, with your knees bent and your feet flat on the mat.

2. Bend your elbows and place your hands on the blanket or bolster, pointing your fingers toward your feet. (You can also squeeze a block between your thighs.)

3. Press down through your legs, lift your hips, and push the wall away from you. Hold this position for 3 to 5 full breaths.

Camel

>>> USTRASANA <<<

This is a kneeling backbend that also doubles as a heart opener, providing you with a gentle stretch in your chest. These movements can also stretch and strengthen your shoulders, abs, and the front of your legs.

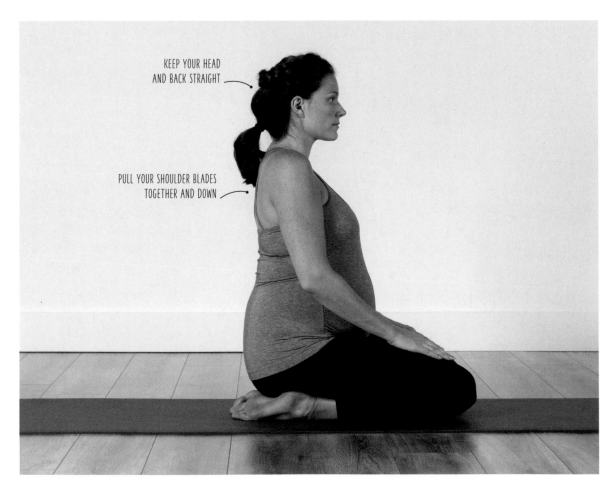

KEEP YOUR HEAD AND BACK STRAIGHT

PULL YOUR SHOULDER BLADES TOGETHER AND DOWN

1 Kneel in the middle of the mat, resting your hands on your knees. Place the tops of your feet flat on the mat.

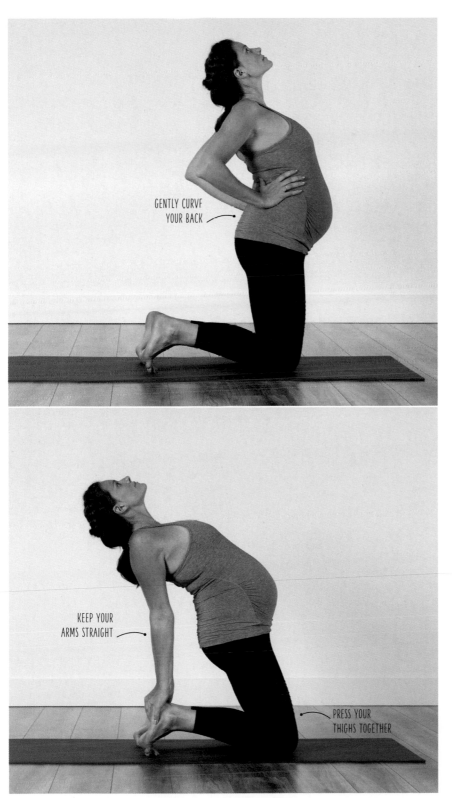

GENTLY CURVE
YOUR BACK

2 Bend your elbows and curl your toes under. Place your hands on your hips and lift your upper chest, shoulders, and head back until you're looking straight up.

KEEP YOUR
ARMS STRAIGHT

PRESS YOUR
THIGHS TOGETHER

3 Extend your arms behind you, grab your heels with your hands, and continue to lean backward, stopping when you've stretched as far as comfortable. (Grab your calves or ankles if that's easier.) Hold this position for 3 to 5 full breaths.

~ CAMEL ~
# VARIATIONS

These variations can help you get over the hump and make the movements of this pose more accessible.

⟨⟨⟨ VARIATION #1

1. Kneel in front of a wall, with your knees flat against the wall and your arms relaxed at your sides. Place blocks short edges up on the outsides of your heels.

2. Press your hips and thighs into the wall. Extend your arms behind you and place your hands on the blocks. Hold this position for 3 to 5 full breaths.

PULL YOUR SHOULDER BLADES TOGETHER AND DOWN

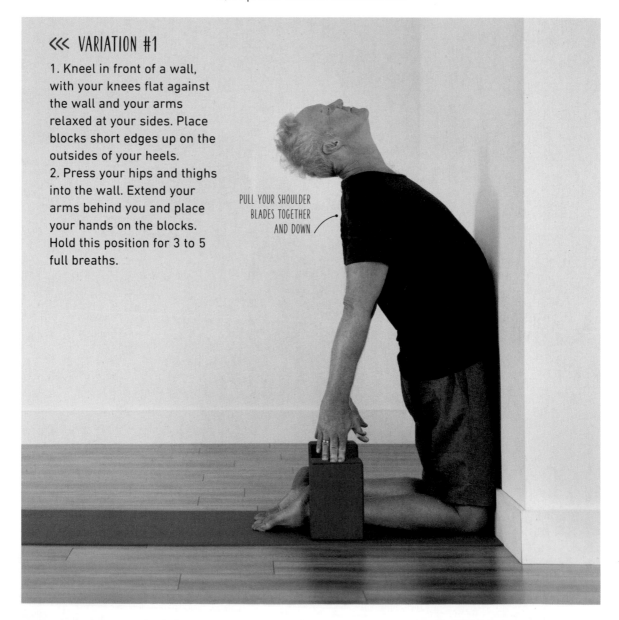

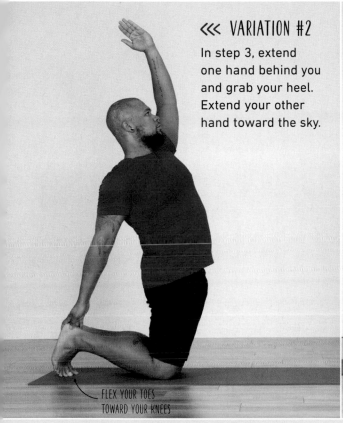

≪ VARIATION #2

In step 3, extend one hand behind you and grab your heel. Extend your other hand toward the sky.

FLEX YOUR TOES TOWARD YOUR KNEES

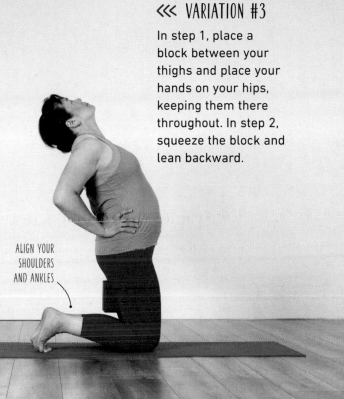

≪ VARIATION #3

In step 1, place a block between your thighs and place your hands on your hips, keeping them there throughout. In step 2, squeeze the block and lean backward.

ALIGN YOUR SHOULDERS AND ANKLES

≪ VARIATION #4

In step 2, place an exercise ball behind your thighs and between your lower legs. (Use one that can comfortably support your body.) In step 3, lean back onto the ball. Rest your arms on the ball, by your sides, or in a prayer position in front of your chest.

KEEP YOUR FEET FLAT ON THE MAT

Legs Up the Wall

>>> VIPARITA KARANI <<<

For this restorative and accessible inversion pose,
you don't need much strength or flexibility. Instead, a wall
allows your body to relax and reset. This is also a great pose
for bringing your breathing back to balance.

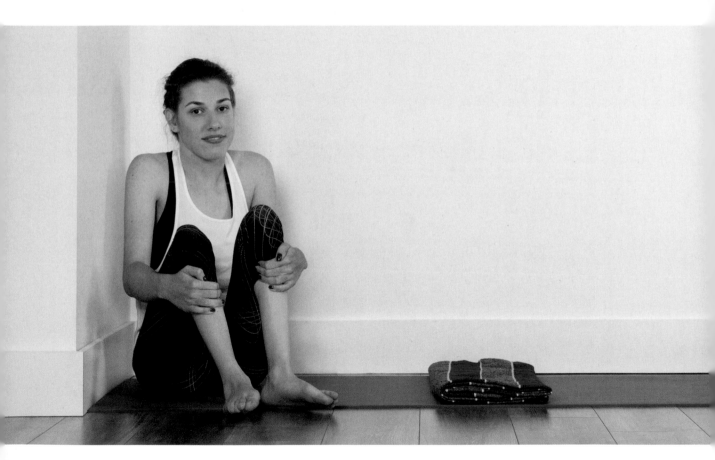

1 Sit with the right side of your body as close to a wall as possible, with your knees bent and your hands resting on your shins.

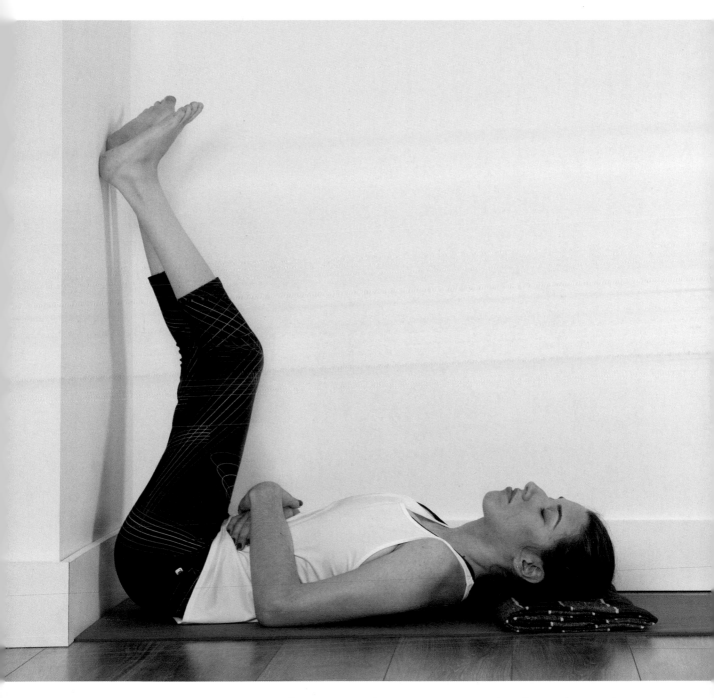

2 Rotate your body to your right and walk your feet up the wall until your body forms an L. Elongate your breathing by taking slow, deep inhales and exhales through your nose. Hold this position for 3 to 5 full breaths. (Adjust these movements as needed to make this a more relaxing pose you're comfortable holding for an extended period of time.)

~ LEGS UP THE WALL ~

VARIATIONS

This pose has many benefits—connecting with your breathing, helping with fatigue, and alleviating swelling in your lower body—but these variations make the movements just a little more accessible.

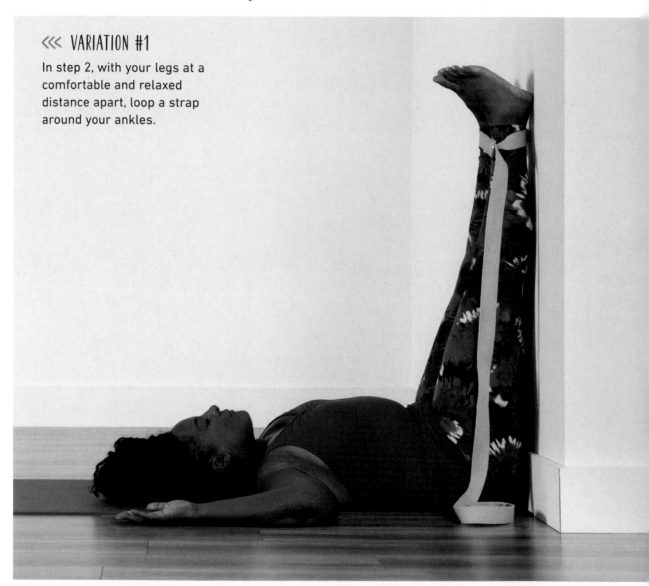

≪ VARIATION #1

In step 2, with your legs at a comfortable and relaxed distance apart, loop a strap around your ankles.

‹‹‹ VARIATION #2

1. Place a chair against a wall, with the seat facing away from the wall and a folded blanket on the seat. Bend your knees and place your legs across the seat of the chair.
2. Slip your feet through the chair and place the balls of your feet flat against the wall. (You can also walk your feet up the back of the chair.) Hold this position for 3 to 5 full breaths.

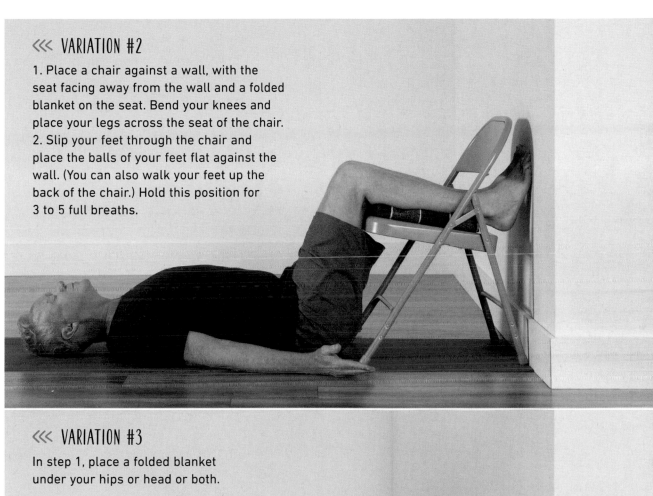

‹‹‹ VARIATION #3

In step 1, place a folded blanket under your hips or head or both.

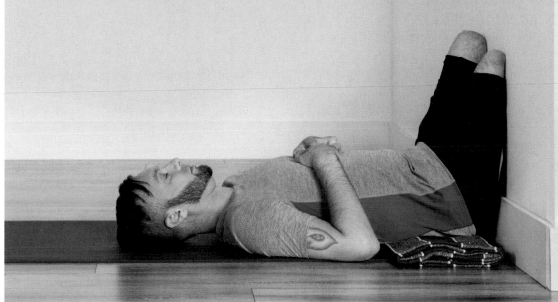

GAIL

WHO IS GAIL PARKER?

I'd describe myself as a trailblazer, pioneer, renegade—courageous, strong, wise, fulfilled, playful, and happy. I've been practicing yoga for 50 years and teaching for 20 years. I'm still learning. That's the power and the gift of yoga. It's the never-ending story.

HOW DID YOU GET STARTED PRACTICING YOGA?

I was introduced to yoga by a master and have been practicing and living yoga ever since. I was 22 years old and curious enough to take a yoga class that was taught at the Detroit Institute of Arts by J. Oliver Black (a.k.a. Yogachraya), one of Paramahansa Yogananda's main disciples. I studied with him for one year and then engaged in a home practice for the next 20 years, as there were no yoga studios in existence and teacher-taught classes were next to impossible to find. To advance, I found books that taught the practices and I studied them.

The emphasis in the yoga I was introduced to was taught as a lifestyle and as a way of thinking, being, and acting, with minimal emphasis on asana and maximum emphasis on self-realization. Once yoga studios began to proliferate, I enthusiastically joined studio classes, eventually took yoga teacher training, and began to integrate yoga philosophy and various practices into my psychotherapy practice. I now teach aspiring yoga therapists and health care providers how to utilize yoga to support emotional health and well-being as self-care practices for themselves and their client populations.

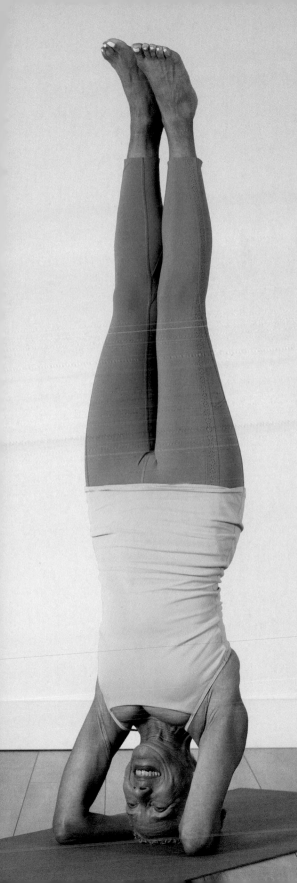

FAVORITE POSE
≫ SUPPORTED HEADSTAND

MOST CHALLENGING POSE
≫ YOGA SQUAT

OCCUPATION
≫ PSYCHOLOGIST, YOGA
EDUCATOR, YOGA THERAPIST

WHAT HAS YOGA HELPED YOU WITH IN YOUR PERSONAL AND PROFESSIONAL LIVES?

I felt empowered by yoga. It shaped my consciousness mentally, emotionally, and spiritually and supported me in making wise choices, including enrolling in graduate school to become a psychologist and leaving a physically and emotionally abusive marriage all within one year of beginning my yoga practice.

I love everything about the practice of yoga physically, emotionally, and spiritually—the yamas, niyamas, asanas, pranayama, and meditation. It has impacted me profoundly personally and professionally, including my pioneering efforts to blend psychology, yoga, and meditation as effective self-care strategies that can enhance emotional balance and contribute to the overall health and well-being of practitioners. I currently have a special interest in utilizing and teaching restorative yoga and meditation as self-care practices for managing ethnic- and race-based stress and trauma.

Look for teachers who live their yoga and who understand and teach yoga as a lifestyle, not just as a physical practice. It might take a few tries to find just the right teacher and just the right practice, but you'll know it when you find it. Don't give up.

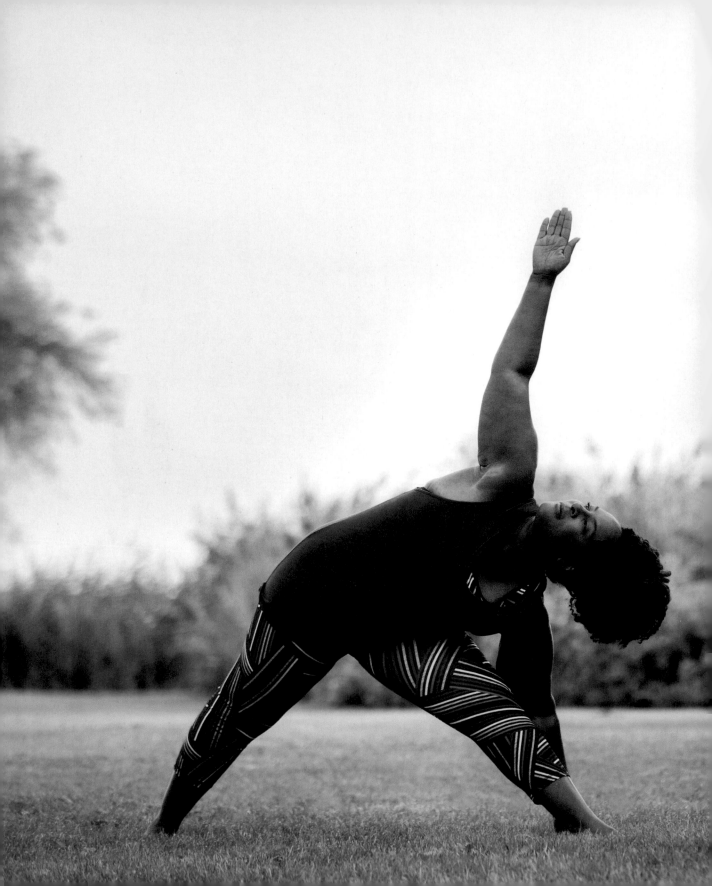

CHAPTER 4

Sequences

This chapter is all about building your personal practice through performing sequences designed to get you started and keep you on the mat. You can practice these sequences when you want, as many times as you like, and at your own pace. You can also enhance your own practice by combining two or more sequences together.

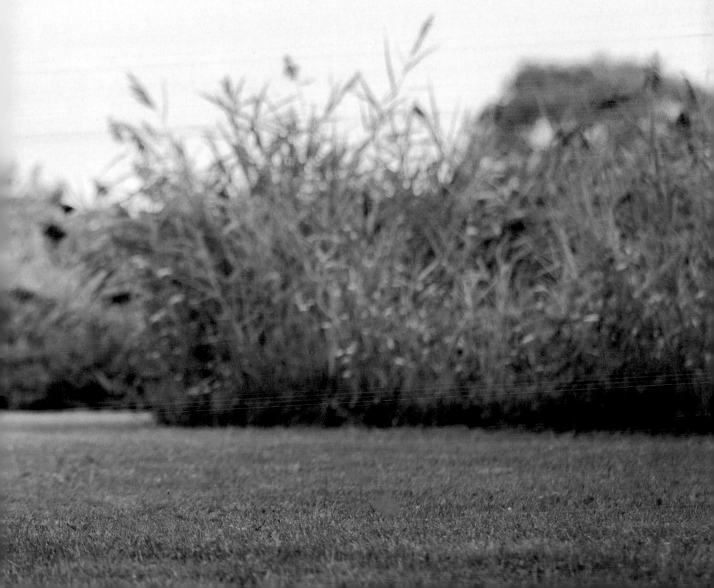

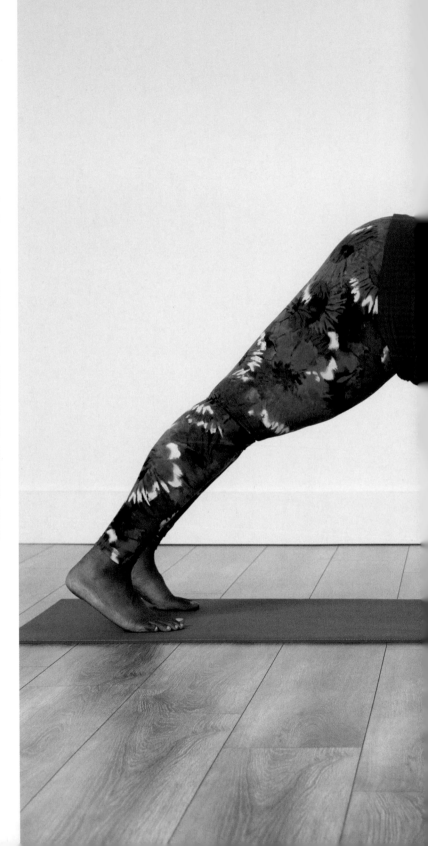

MORNING PRACTICE

This sequence is all about energizing you for taking on the day and whatever it brings. These poses are also great for helping you center your breathing.

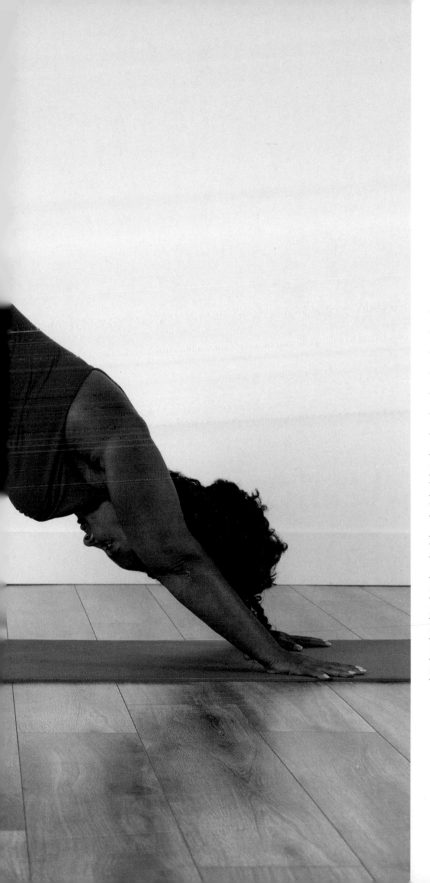

SUN SALUTATION

Reset, reboot, and rejuvenate
your energy with the poses
in this sequence—all in praise
of the star that brings us light
and enlightenment.

BEDTIME PRACTICE

No time during the day is a bad time for yoga, and this sequence will prove that. These poses can help you unwind from the day and get ready for bed.

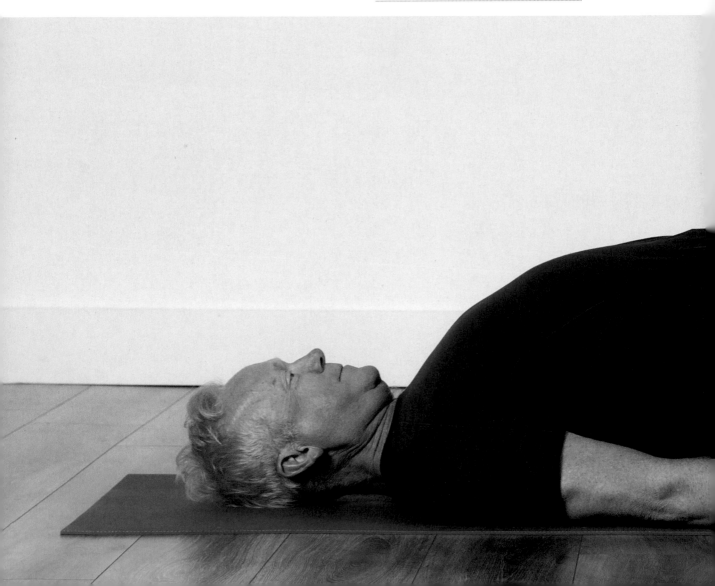

EASING BACK PAIN

If you suffer from back pain, this sequence can offer some relief. And if you already have a strong back, these poses can help enhance that strength.

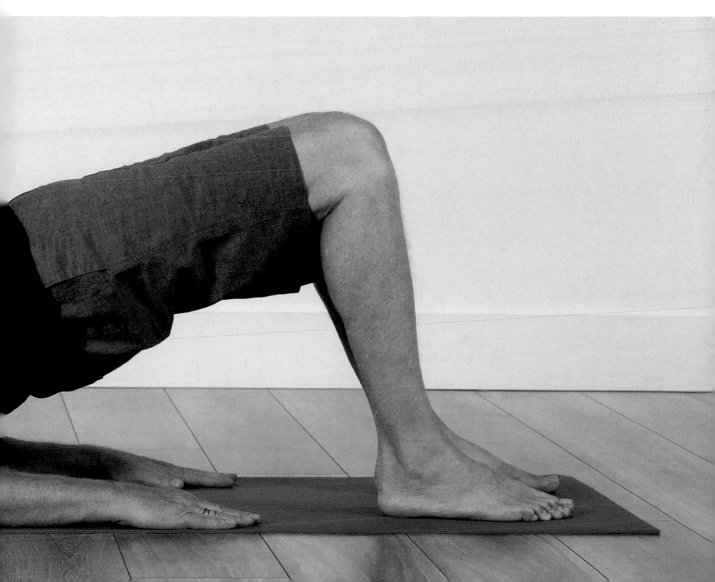

IMPROVING FLEXIBILITY

Not only can these poses help you increase your flexibility, but they can also enhance the range of motion in your joints. Practicing this sequence can ease achiness, pain, and stiffness in muscles and joints.

FINDING BALANCE

We're always seeking balance—physical, mental, emotional, and spiritual—and your yoga practice can help you reach a place of calm and contentment. That's what these poses are all about.

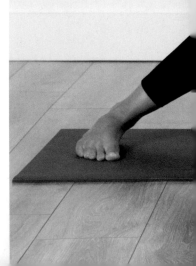

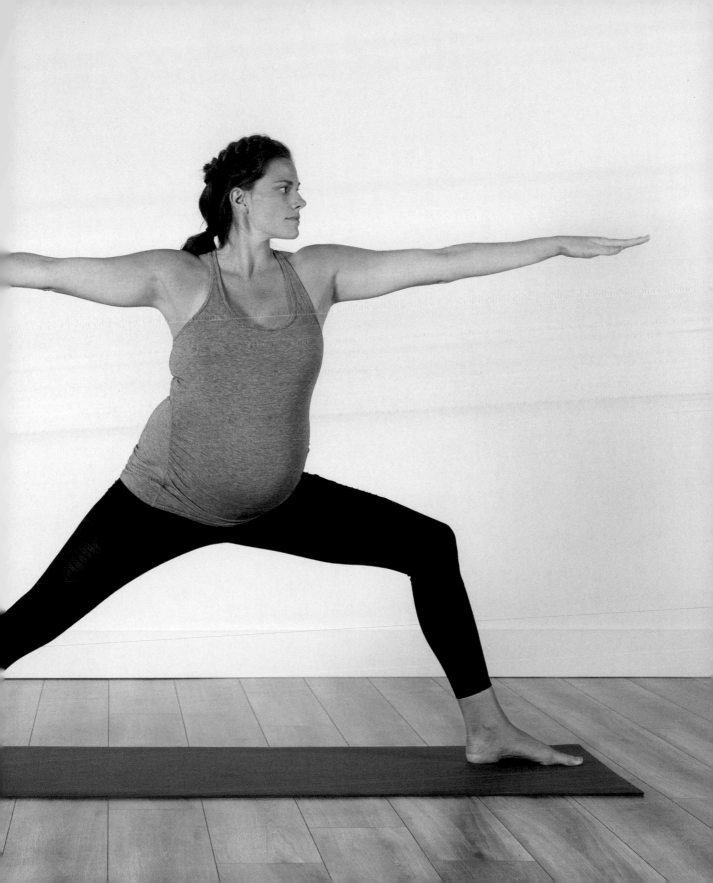

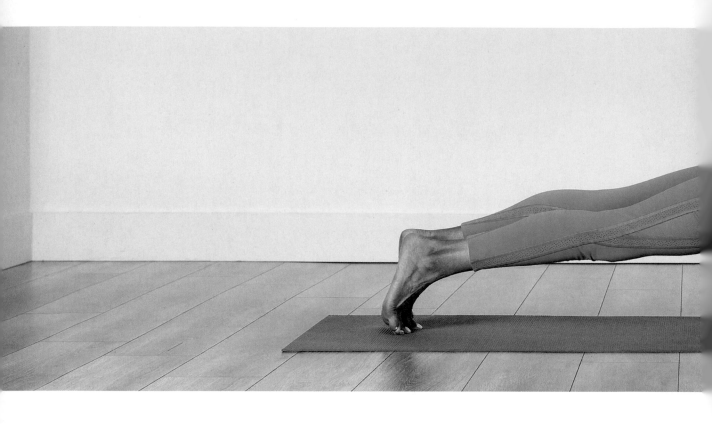

BUILDING STRENGTH

Reaching a state of physical and mental stability can help you with almost any everyday task. These poses can help bring you closer to that stability.

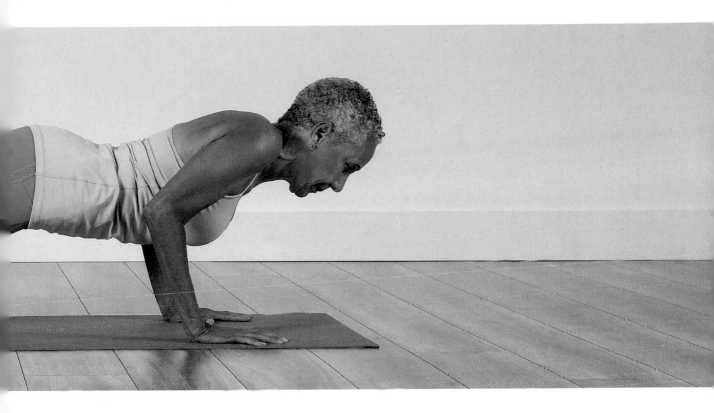

STRENGTHENING CORE

Your core muscles are critical for many everyday motions, including extending, bending, and twisting. These poses can help you strengthen these muscles.

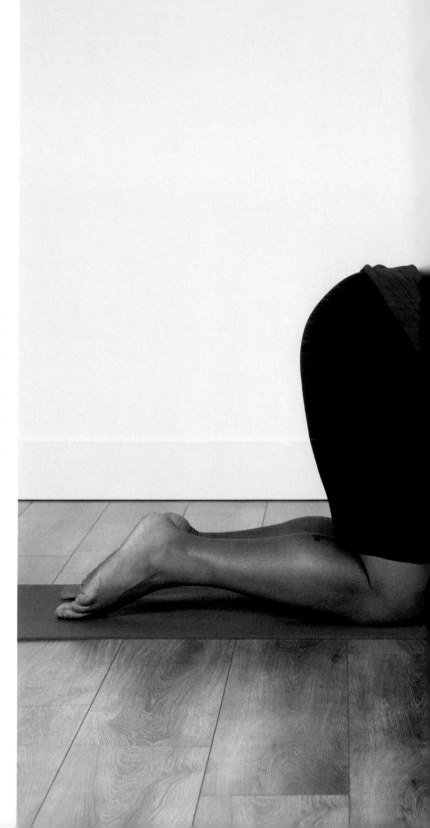

RELIEVING STRESS

Stress can negatively impact
and influence our everyday actions.
But practicing this sequence can
help you focus on what you need
to do to tame that wild stress.

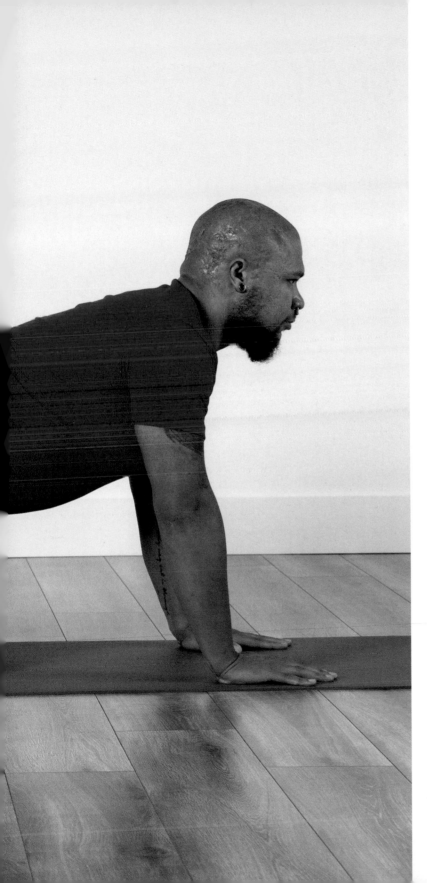

YOGA AT THE WALL

All these poses come with
a variation that involves a chair.
You'll be surprised at how much
you gain physically and mentally
by practicing yoga while sitting.

Index

ABOUT THE AUTHOR

Dianne Bondy is a yoga teacher who's a leading voice of the Yoga for All movement. Her views about yoga empower thousands of practitioners around the world—regardless of shape, size, ethnicity, or ability. Dianne contributes to *Yoga International* magazine and the Do You Yoga initiative. She's also been featured by several international media outlets, including *The Guardian*, *Huffington Post*, *Cosmopolitan*, *People*, *ESPN*, and more. Dianne is a leading spokesperson for diversity in yoga, as showcased by her affiliations with Accessible Yoga, Gaiam, and the Yoga & Body Image Coalition. Her writings have been published in *Yoga and Body Image* and *Yes Yoga Has Curves*.

ACKNOWLEDGMENTS

Writing this book was important to me. I want to thank all the people who trusted me with their practice. I want to acknowledge that people from all walks of life can do yoga. We can shape the poses to fit our bodies and help us connect with our breath.

I'm grateful to be given the opportunity to share yoga more inclusively. First off, I want to thank my mom for sharing this practice with me at a young age. I would like to thank Alan, my partner, for supporting my journey. To Cristina Matteis, Beth Reidy, and Juliane Spriet, thanks for all your assistance, guidance, and support in helping me clarify words and my teachings for this book so I can share this knowledge with everyone.

PUBLISHER'S ACKNOWLEDGMENTS

The publisher wishes to thank Alexandra, Don, Dylan, Gail, Gwen, John, Josie, and especially Dianne for being models for this book. We couldn't have created this book without you. You're aspirational and inspirational!